The Far Side of the Moon

Also by Clive Stafford Smith

Injustice: Life and Death in the Courtrooms of America
Bad Men: Guantánamo Bay and the Secret Prisons

Falkirk Council

Meadowbank Library
2a Stevenson Avenue
Polmont
FK2 0GU

Bo'ness
01506 778520

Bonnybridge
01324 503295

Denny
01324 504242

Falkirk
01324 503605

Grangemouth
01324 504690

Larbert
01324 503590

Meadowbank
01324 503870

Slamannan
01324 851373

This book is due
for return on or
before the last date
indicated on the
label. Renewals
may be obtained
on application.

Clive Stafford Smith

The Far Side of the Moon

Trials of My Father

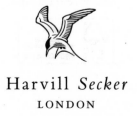

Harvill *Secker*

LONDON

1 3 5 7 9 10 8 6 4 2

Harvill Secker, an imprint of Vintage, is part of the Penguin Random House group of companies whose addresses can be found at global.penguinrandom-house.com

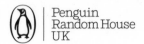

First published by Harvill Secker in 2022

penguin.co.uk/vintage

A CIP catalogue record for this book is available from the British Library

ISBN 9781787301924 (hardback)

Typeset in 11.5/15 pt Bembo by Jouve (UK), Milton Keynes
Printed and bound in Great Britain by Clays Ltd, Elcograf S.p.A.

The authorised representative in the EEA is Penguin Random House Ireland, Morrison Chambers, 32 Nassau Street, Dublin D02 Y H68

Penguin Rand[...] House is committed to a sustainable future for [o]ur business, our readers [...] This book is made from Fore[st] Ste[...]rdship Council® certified paper.

This book is dedicated to our mother, Jean Stafford Smith, who always put herself between us and harm.

CONTENTS

The Far Side of the Moon

Introduction: Getting Angry

I need not therefore make any doubt of Melancholy, but that it is an hereditary disease.

Robert Burton, *The Anatomy of Melancholy*

I got truly angry with Dad for the first time in 2017. By then, he had been dead for a little over ten years, so I was a bit late. Prior to that, I had felt varied emotions over the years. When I was very young his enthusiasm inspired me and my friends. He could be the perfect dad, brilliant and challenging. A little later came the confusion: for example, he told me, at the age of seven, that it was time for me to leave home and make my own way in the world. I didn't understand why he would say or write something quite kind about me one day, and within twenty-four hours be telling the world I was the spawn of Satan. My older brother, Mark, and sister, Mary, were treated similarly. As I began to understand that Dad was unwell, I felt sympathy and – far worse – pity for him.

The nadir came in my thirties when I found him boring. He would go on and on about his latest idea, which I knew from experience would crash and burn, signifying nothing.

I don't remember being angry at him when he was alive. Maybe I wasn't allowed that emotion until long after he was dead.

As a sixteen-year-old, I read about people on death row, and it seemed extraordinary that a contemporary government would conduct some form of human sacrifice to a mythological god of deterrence. This led me to a youthful ambition to go to university in the US, with the notion that I would write the seminal book on the iniquities of capital punishment. With an astounding arrogance, I thought my book could persuade the US to mend its ways. My gradual awakening from this grandiosity began when I spent six months visiting condemned prisoners in Georgia, and learned that they had a rather more pressing need for legal assistance than for a book that nobody would read. So I went to law school instead, with my completed manuscript (*Life on Death Row*) preserved only for the amusement of future grandchildren.

When I began representing prisoners under death sentence, with all their diverse frailties, I soon learned that my job was to figure out what made people tick – and often what led them to murder. I got quite adept at working out my clients' full stories, and even sharing their paths with relatives of the victims, who had a mighty motive to hate the perpetrator. I had my share of failures along the way, but my clients taught me some of life's basic rules: people must feel empathy, rather than pity or even sympathy, if they are to be open-hearted. Pitying the prisoners sets them apart; empathy makes us see them as human.

I encountered many people who suffered from 'mental illness', in all the guises described in the diagnostic manual. I fear I will put mental illness in inverted commas whenever the term raises its head for a number of reasons. First, the very concept is a large part of the stigma that my father, along with so many others, had to live with. Second, the distinction between things mental and physical is dubious and is, I believe, rooted in a very human insecurity, a notion that we somehow elevate ourselves by tearing down the animal kingdom and consigning them to an inferior species. And third, as we will discuss, there is the principle so brilliantly elucidated in Isaac Asimov's book *I, Robot* seventy years ago – or by Will Smith in the movie rather more recently: the notion that the human brain is more than a fantastically complex and interesting series of electronic impulses is rather silly.

But enough of that for now. Dad was described as bipolar,

and a few of my clients were labelled in the same way. I had been living on the edges of Dad's 'illness' for most of my life, yet I had only the barest comprehension of what having such an 'illness' meant. Indeed, I fled from him as far as I could, going to America when I was still a teenager. In due course, my elder siblings Mark and Mary both went to Australia. All three of us were keen to create some genetic distance as well. We were sitting together one time, and Mark expressed a concern that he might 'turn out' like Dad – the one to inherit the bipolar gene. Mary burst out laughing; even I managed a smile. Mary said it was obvious to anyone with eyes to see that I was our father's child, not Mark. Indeed, I already had an agreement with Mary: if I were to go Dad's way, I would trust her to get me into a psychiatric hospital, even against my will, to make sure I got treatment. But I did not comprehend much more about Dad, or about myself; in retrospect, I am not sure any of us did.

After twenty-six years in the US, I headed back to England in 2004, in part because both of my parents were ageing. Dad died in 2007 when I was in Mauritania on a Guantánamo Bay case. As usual I put my client before my father – or else I would have rescheduled the trip. Dad had just been moved from Addenbrooke's Hospital in Cambridge to a residential home. I visited him briefly, finding him in a Dickensian atmosphere, with demented patients howling like caged beasts. Horrified, I resolved to move him as soon as I returned, but I took my flight to the Mauritanian capital, Nouakchott, anyway. I heard about his death by phone, as I watched the stars over the Sahara Desert from a hotel balcony.

He was the dad I had; my guide, for good and for ill, when it came to being a father myself. At his funeral, I resolved, belatedly, to write a book about him, to help myself see why his life had been so unhappy. But not yet. My aunt – Dad's elder sister, Jean – used to get upset when I talked about his 'illness'. She had suffered more than anyone from his poisoned pen and razor tongue and did not deserve to have me resurrecting the vampires of her life. She joked her way stoically through a rapidly swelling throat cancer, and died in 2015.

That was when I set about Dad in earnest. My mother had kept many documents, including 3,000 of his letters (he was more manic than depressed). I read them and took close notes. Many of the documents were new to me. Mum had supported him through the thick and mostly thin of his life, even for the thirty-five years after she had the good sense to divorce him. I had been in the US for much of that time, and I discovered that for me she had censored the spleen that spewed out in the cycle that steadily alienated him from the world. There was even an article in the *Newmarket Journal* that I had never seen before in which he had advocated my immediate execution.

That which I had not known had not hurt me, and it was clearly evidence that he was manic at the time. Yet such very public laundering of our family issues must have been horrendous for my mother, whose neighbours would all have subscribed to the local paper. Then there were the scores of letters in which Dad had aimed his angst at her and my aunt. But what hurt my mother most was when he attacked one of her children; then she would respond, crisply and with great sense.

Even though, intellectually, I could see that his 'illness' was the author of the venomous words, I found it difficult to avoid an anger I had never previously felt.

I was also very sad. He had had such potential and it had come to so very little.

Around the time Dad was advocating my electrocution, I was spending a large proportion of my time trying to save the life of Larry Lonchar, who was on death row in Georgia. We find the teeth to fit our wounds and Larry served as a surrogate for Dad – not in the sense of parenting, but because he also suffered from bipolar disorder. His life ran parallel with Dad's in various ways. Each was put into a coma by a passing car at an early age, with an imponderable impact on their later lives. Dad had a complex relationship with his parents – there was his Jewish anti-Semitic mother, obsessed by the nouveau riche status she gained when her husband, Albert, inherited Cheveley Park Stud from his former employer, Robert Sherwood. Larry similarly 'inherited' a difficult set of parents: alcoholics whose pathology blinded them to their son's problems.

Dad graduated from private school to RAF Bomber Command when still sixteen – his mother could never say no to him, and falsified his birth certificate. His subsequent trauma scarred him in ways that are difficult for my generation to fathom. Larry, from his early teens, was also dispatched by his mother to join an institution – reform school, followed later by prison – where he could scrape at the scabs left by his family.

The only way Larry could make money in prison was to gamble with increasing recklessness. Dad gambled any money he had away, in the throes of his mania. Larry was seen as nothing more than a criminal, just as the world saw Dad as a spendthrift and a fraud. Ultimately, in their depressive phases, they both saw themselves as worthless.

In some ways, though, the two of them were inverted images. Dad was more manic than depressed and, to my knowledge, only once seriously considered taking his own life; Larry was more often depressed, and would periodically drop his appeals in order to effect suicide by electric chair. He came within forty minutes of death three times – somehow a court would block it. The fourth time, it was the end of the eleventh hour: the Supreme Court issued a stay with a mere fifty-eight seconds left on the clock.

Sad to say, I ignored Dad for much of my life. Even with Larry I was too busy trying to walk him back from death to understand him, let alone figure out whether he was actually guilty of the crime. Instead, I pinned the same label on him as I did my dad. I was focused on each as a problem, as 'bipolar'.

The concept of 'mental illness' carries with it a heavy burden. Dad himself would rather have been seen as Bad than Mad – though he imagined he was neither. The state of Georgia was very keen to see Larry as Bad, and Larry saw himself that way long before the government branded him a killer.

There is a circular track to some lives, where the runners keep doing laps, getting nowhere nearer to any destination, only becoming exhausted. They find themselves on the outside of our community, looking in. We think they should adapt to our structure; they can't. This alienates them further. Their behaviour becomes more extreme, and the cycle continues.

Dad inherited Cheveley Park Stud, famous in the world of horse racing, from his father. Nobody ever paused to consider whether he was suited to a profession that revolves entirely around gambling – from how the sperm of the stallion and the egg of the mare will coalesce, to how the foal will eventually adapt to a damp racetrack at Newbury with an irascible jockey on board. Dad was too impatient for such a complex and long-term project. He drove the stud into bankruptcy in a swirl of inevitability.

Larry's fate was on a parallel path, albeit to a verdict for triple murder rather than bankruptcy. As the two of them blundered through life, frustrated at each turn, they drove away all those around them until they found themselves alone, and intensely lonely. Neither was inclined to accept 'treatment' for his 'illness'.

In this book, I wonder whether we might map out a plan by which everything could have been different. First, we might do away with most of our notions of 'mental illness', which are often shorthand for our lack of understanding. If we were talking about a physical 'disability' the approach would seem obvious to us all: we would not tell someone in a wheelchair to stand up and play basketball like Michael Jordan; we would see how we could adapt the game to fit their disability (or better yet, their ability).

Why do we not take a similar approach with 'mental' issues? Dad found himself in a career chosen by inheritance rather than aligned with his idiosyncrasies. Mania does not mesh well with our nine-to-five world: Dad would happily work from 3 a.m. to midnight and, while that might seem productive, if nobody else operated on the same schedule he was doomed to disappointment. He might have had a great idea, but he could never hang around to see it implemented.

My studies over the years suggested that there were some occupations that were ideally suited to his nature. For example – and here I am truly oversimplifying the issue – Vincent van Gogh failed in his early career as an art dealer, but as a painter he could press on all day and all night if he wanted to, without troubling anyone (though he should have been dissuaded from cutting his ear off). Similarly, Dad was a fine poet, and the arts were much better suited to his temperament than running a business was.

There are practicalities that we must take into account. To the argument that Dad could not have made a living as a poet, the response might be that he never made a living at anything else either. He was fortunate that our immediate family supported him financially for most of his life, though sometimes he resented it (he had been indoctrinated to believe that he had to be the breadwinner). I, for one, never thought about his vocation until it was much too late.

Society likes to draw a distinction between the 'physical' and the 'mental', partly due to our penchant for holding people 'responsible' for their actions. We posit concepts like the 'soul' or the 'conscience' and say that people make choices, but we do this more to justify punishing them than to cherish their creativity. Perhaps the notion of a 'soul' and its happy elevation to a heaven is, as Stephen Hawking once suggested, a confection for those who are afraid of the dark. Perhaps we will gradually accept that we do not diminish our respect for each other, and for the magnificent complexity of humanity, by seeking mitigation in all those who behave badly. Perhaps as we gradually develop greater understanding, we will see that there is a precipitant for everything that any person does; whether we want to call it an excuse, an explanation, or the trait of an 'evil character' depends on how unkind we wish to be. It also, perhaps, depends on whether we want to seek a solution or simply cast blame.

That said, we cannot solve every problem by wishing it away or moving the goalposts. Sometimes, life insists on a paradox. Larry presented a different challenge from my father, and like all of us, he lived in a world where people can be simply cruel. Of course, many would say that he was brutal himself, assuming that he really did take part in a triple homicide. I came to love his warped humanity. Dad could truly have been a poet, but Larry was not going to be permitted the life he would really wish for. The best he might expect was an acceptable prison.

In writing about Dad and Larry, I hope to explore how we could, at least, remove some of the stigma that dogged them. By the time he had driven his family and friends away, Larry was in an isolation cell surrounded by guards who wanted to kill him – who wouldn't become even more depressed? Likewise, one Christmas, late in his life, Dad found that only his Dictaphone would listen to his circular self-justifications – who wouldn't be lonely?

Much too late to be of much use to either Dad or Larry, I sat down to try to work out what went so terribly wrong in their lives, and how it might have gone better. I am not sure I have many of the answers, but I hope I can begin a conversation with those who care to read it, and perhaps edge a little closer to understanding what we really mean by 'mental illness'.

Meanwhile, I belatedly worked out that I could not expect to destigmatise their situations if I did not recognise that I, too, am well along their spectrum. I have to look in the mirror from time to time, to avoid rendering Dad and Larry as animals in a zoo. I also should have spent less time trying to control Dad and Larry, and more on identifying the passions that made their lives meaningful.

Dad and Larry both died before I figured this out. If Dad's belief in reincarnation was justified, he has come back in a happier form. I doubt it. If Larry's faith held any truth, he is now in heaven. Again, I suspect that dust is once again dust.

Those of us who remain can, however, hope to make a little less of a hash of things with the next generation.

1

Great-Granny Frances Canham: Sending Back Soiled Goods

> What passing-bells for these who die as cattle?
>> Wilfred Owen, 'Anthem for Doomed Youth'

Dad never met his grandmother Frances Canham, though she did not die until he was ten. Frances was one of my family's many hidden secrets.

Her husband, Daniel Whisker, was born in 1859, exactly a hundred years before me. He was a saddler, originally from Bow, in London. After ten years making saddles for the ladies and gentlemen riding gently around Hyde Park, he moved to Newmarket, the world capital of racing. Daniel's ambition was to create the strongest, lightest saddles to help jockeys and trainers claim the great prizes of the track. He invented the first one-pound racing saddle, whereupon he felt he was ready for marriage. In 1890, he met Frances Sarah Canham, vivacious and eight years his junior. They were married on 23 November 1891, and he moved from his digs into Allington House on the high street. Two years later, they had their first child, Beatrix, my grandmother. Trix was followed by Ve in 1896, and Edgar just as the century turned.

A fourth child, Freda, died in infancy, with a devastating impact on Frances. She was first depressed – 'melancholic' was the word used at the time – before she fell victim to another burden of marriage a century ago: there were only rudimentary methods of contraception, and Frances was forty-four when she gave birth to Joan just before Christmas 1911.

Fulbourn Hospital, on the outskirts of Cambridge, has made episodic interventions in my family history. It opened its doors as Fulbourn Asylum in 1858. Frances found herself there early in 1912. She was, it seems, carrying the family defect.

It was the age of eugenics. 'Prevention of the increase of insanity,' Fulbourn's superintendent, Dr Thompson, wrote, 'will be brought about by the legal control and segregation of the unfit, so that defectives will not be added to the community.' Dr Thompson was a tyrant, still remembered decades later by residents of the asylum for holding a fire drill in the middle of Christmas dinner, causing all the food to spoil.

The records for Fulbourn Asylum are held in the Cambridge archives. A disproportionate number of Fulbourn's inmates were Frances's soulmates, diagnosed with chronic post-natal mania or melancholia. Justice for the 'mentally ill' varied wildly, yet there were seeds of hope. In 1911, Rose Doubleday, a woman 'with no employment', was sectioned for 'volitional insanity' – the act of stealing was madness. She was said to have 'recovered' six months later, conveniently the precise length of what would otherwise have been a criminal sentence. Rose's treatment suggested that the early twentieth century was moving in a compassionate direction, viewing antisocial behaviour as 'mental abnormality' rather than as 'evil'.

Frances was soon shipped to another asylum in London, near to her parents. She spent twenty-four years at Peckham House Asylum, 'a Metropolitan Licensed Mad House', where the records speak of brutality and a diet of meagre portions of watery soup and stale bread. She was far away from her four children in Newmarket, and consigned to abject conditions until she finally died in 1935, at the age of sixty-eight.

I wondered whether this was all her husband could manage, as he was already in his fifties when she was sectioned, and he now had four children to care for on his own. I checked out his will from the records in Ipswich: he died a year earlier than

Frances, on 14 April 1934, leaving £4,854 – the equivalent of over £300,000 today. He had become a wealthy master saddler, but he had hidden his wife in a paupers' asylum.

The eldest daughter, Trix, would have been eighteen when her mother was sectioned. She was the one saddled with her three younger siblings, including the infant Joan. But her mother's fate was not the only 'embarrassment' Trix hid. For one, she was Jewish via both her parents, something so well disguised that I did not learn my father was Jewish until I was forty – twenty years after I had joined a Jewish fraternity in my American university, thinking I was the statutory goy. Trix was also ashamed of her economic status. Flat racing was the sport of queens: only people with the wealth of a monarch could afford to own racehorses. The stud owner came next in the hierarchy, and then the trainer: even though either may have owned significant property, both were beholden to the horse owner. Jockeys might be stars, respected for their talent, yet they were either privileged amateurs or working professionals. Further down yet, Trix's father, Daniel, was a *tradesman*. Trix could not abide this; she was a snob, which meant, sadly, that she hated everything about herself.

In 1917, she set her sights on Albert Smith. His forebears had, like hers, fled the pogroms in Russia, though he also kept his ethnicity well hidden under his English pseudonym. I never met my grandfather as he died in 1958, the year before I was born. He was a distant man, apparently, but I suspect I would have liked him. He had come upon something of an education, and in his early twenties he arrived in Newmarket from Worksop to work as the personal secretary to Robert Louis Vodoz Sherwood, who owned a training stable at St Gatien House, named after his 1884 Derby winner – actually the only true dead heat in Derby history.

Albert was a pacifist. When the Great War began he was twenty-seven but, unlike so many of his generation, he did not rush to sign up. He continued his work for Mr Sherwood until

December 1915, when the government finally caught up with him. He joined the Army Reserve as an ambulance driver, but was fortunate to develop appendicitis, which kept him off duty for a year. In 1917, however, he found himself on the Italian front. He was not required to kill, but he had to witness a great deal of senseless death. I came across pages torn from his diary for the year, filled with his pencil jottings. The Italian trenches are less well known than those of Ypres or the Somme, but they were equally drenched in blood. All in all, there were, for example, *twelve* fruitless battles of the Isonzo. On 12 May 1917, following infinitesimal gains made in the first nine, the Italians directed a two-pronged attack against Austrian forces north and east of Gorizia in the Tenth Battle of the Isonzo. They managed to break through and capture the Banjšice Plateau. Finding themselves on the verge of victory, their supply lines could not keep up and they were forced to withdraw.

Albert retreated with them, leaving many bodies behind. For two weeks, he did no more than tick off each day as he simply survived. 'Bad night,' he noted. 'An explosion nearly blew me out of bed. It was an ammunition train. Another air raid came quite close to the house.' On 16 July the neighbouring village was bombed, with forty killed and sixty injured. As the ambulance driver, he descended into the midst of it all.

'Still in bed and feeling absolutely run down,' he scrawled two mornings later. 'Went over to Villa to see Doctor Brock . . . he says it is all nerves.' Albert was suffering from shell shock – today we call it post-traumatic stress disorder, or PTSD.

By August 1917, the eleventh futile Battle of the Isonzo had begun. Mutinies and plummeting morale crippled the Italian Army. Then Albert found himself in the twelfth Battle of the Isonzo: through all twelve battles, casualties along the river were enormous – more than a quarter of a million men. Fortunately, he had home leave for the second time in the war. He felt his mortality during these times, and he proposed to Trix, was accepted, and they were married on 15 August 1918. At the time, nobody was sure how long this war would last. However, by the end of October, the Austro-Hungarian Empire was falling apart. Czechoslovakia, Croatia and Slovenia proclaimed their independence, and troops started deserting. Italy assembled enough soldiers to mount an offensive and broke through near Sacile, crushing the Austrian defensive line. The Austrian government sued for peace, which was concluded on 3 November.

By this time Albert Smith was on his way home. He had survived the carnage, intact in body if not entirely in spirit.

When he returned to Newmarket, Albert was once again personal secretary to Bob Sherwood, and they became very close friends. (How close, Dad only worked out seventy-five years later.) The older Sherwood, Robert Sr, had been a trainer, and an amateur jockey before that. Bob was an only child, a racing friend of Winston Churchill. Indeed, when I was growing up we had every meal at Churchill's old dining table. Robert Sr had been a millionaire in today's money, and when Bob came into his inheritance in 1921, he decided to move up a Newmarket class, from trainer to breeder. He bought Cheveley Park Stud, the magnificent racing establishment with a pedigree for breeding horses going back 997 years to the time of King Athelstan in 924, and owned by kings from Canute to Edward II. The stud had trees to match: Garden House, where I grew up, was shaded by several cedar trees that were listed in the 1086 Domesday Book. They later stood guard over the rather unimpressive Cheveley Castle, built by Sir John de Pulteney in 1347.

By 1624, Cheveley Park had its own racetrack. A terrace near our house, patterned on Versailles, was later added for spectators. Royalty sometimes attended, and there was a grove just inside the far curve of the circuit where the other horses could slow down, out of sight, to allow the Prince of Wales's horse to emerge ahead. The estate passed to the Dukes of Rutland, and John Manners, the 5th Duke, put the stud firmly on the equine map by breeding four winners of Classics races.

The stud reached its apogee in 1892 when it was sold to Colonel Harry McCalmont, who had just acquired a great deal of money from his great-uncle. In the brief fireworks of his life as a millionaire, McCalmont owned Isinglass, one of the most famous thoroughbreds of all time. Between 1892 and 1895, Isinglass won more money in real terms than any other horse in history. McCalmont constructed a home befitting the animal, not so much a stable as a house. There was a door above the horse from which a servant could check on him during the night, should he whinny.

McCalmont had a great Ozymandias project, Cheveley Mansion, which was completed in 1898. It boasted forty-three bedrooms, and one window for each day of the year. He laid a railway up from Newmarket to deliver the materials he needed. He insisted on a real tennis court – which was never used, not even once. Then he went to South Africa with his regiment, returned to London in 1902 and promptly died, aged forty-one, of a heart attack.

Isinglass passed away nine years later, a few months before my great-grandmother Frances suffered her nervous breakdown; his skeleton was gifted to the Natural History Museum, where he remains today. The mansion was briefly used as a hospital in the Great War, before Bob Sherwood spent his inheritance on the stud's three hundred acres. One of the first things he did was demolish the huge house, just twenty-three years after it had been finished.

I don't suppose anyone who knew Granny Trix could imagine her empathising with her husband or his experiences in Italy. Neither did she have much time for her first child, Jean, who was born on 6 November 1920. My aunt Jean was delightful: clever, caustic, she might have had a bright future, if only she had been born either male or fifty years later. But in the 1920s, with a mother who was not interested in the lot of women, Jean had little chance to develop her talents. My father

Richard – known as Dick – was born on 30 August 1925. In the early days, Dad found himself in a family that was still only aspiring to be middle-class. They lived in a house called Doonside, across from the Newmarket tennis courts.

'When Mum told Dick to do something, he just would not do it,' Auntie Jean recalled. 'But if he asked her for something and she said "No", he would keep at her until she said "Yes". In the end, I think whenever anyone said "No", he only ever heard "Yes". That was part of the problem we had.'

Dad was told he had to go to school, and he hated that. At five years old, it may have been the first time in his young life he had encountered discipline, and he ran away. His chosen escape route took him out in front of a car that could not stop and he was in a coma for several days. Facing her brother's manic antics later in life, Auntie Jean used to wonder out loud whether this head injury was the cause of what was to come.

When Trix's father Daniel died in 1934, he left half of his fortune to his son Edgar, and half to Albert. The family jumped up a social notch. Dad went to the Perse in Cambridge, a private day school. Jean never got that chance.

Albert spent his days working closely with his boss, Bob Sherwood, and his evenings at the Roisterer Club in town. In the summer holidays, the family would evacuate to Cromer, on the Norfolk coast. Albert would drive Trix and the two children seventy miles there, and leave them for two months while he returned to Newmarket. When Bob Sherwood died in 1942, unmarried, he left his entire fortune to Albert. Now my family leapfrogged several more rungs in Newmarket society. Albert and Trix immediately moved into the grand old house, St Gatien, and Albert found himself promoted from secretary to stud owner. Trix found herself dining off bone china, and wearing a mink coat.

Cromer was significant to me as well, as we spent our summer holidays there when I was growing up, at the seaside home my parents had bought. In the winter of 2000, my wife Emily and I took Dad up there for auld lang syne. He was then seventy-five and not capable of the long walks we once took, so we pottered down to the pub on the front, where we sat each nursing a drink. It was then that Dad suddenly came out with the fact that both his parents had been Jewish. I was taken aback. Until then, all I had known of my family was the uninteresting family tree on my mother's side, pieced together by my godfather Jeremy, every one of them a Saxon peasant. I pondered Dad's revelation, rather pleased, only vaguely listening as he and Emily continued their conversation.

Dad described how his father would simply dump them in Cromer for months at a time and rarely visit them. Dad loved his beach holidays, but he could not understand his father's total absence. Emily wondered, in turn, how it was that Albert had inherited everything from Bob Sherwood, a man who had blood relatives with first call on his wealth. She was suddenly struck by a possible answer.

'Dick!' she exclaimed. 'I've worked it out! Your father was having a gay relationship with Bob. That's it! It has to be that . . .'

My first thought was that Dad was going to explode. He liked Em and was normally very gallant with her, but her remark had gone well over the solid line of his homophobia. There was a long silence while Dad observed the spume-head on his beer. Eventually he looked up, his eyes moonlike through his NHS glasses.

'Do you know . . . maybe you have a point . . .' he said, to my astonishment. There was an extended pause before he continued. 'I will never forget, at his funeral, his best friend came up to me . . .' He marshalled his own thoughts from 1958. '. . . and said, "Dick, I hope you'll be more of a man than your father was." I've wondered for forty years what on earth he meant. Maybe that was it!'

He and Emily went off on their chitter-chatter, while I was left with my evolving view of my own family: how my

Jewish anti-Semitic grandmother may have been married to a gay Jew, and how this must have impacted on her and my father. Dad might only have just been coming to the party now, but he had to have known something was going on; my enquiries around Newmarket's elderly residents later confirmed that Albert's relationship with Sherwood had been an open secret.

2

Inheriting Post-traumatic Stress Disorder

> I am the enemy you killed, my friend.
> I knew you in this dark: for so you frowned.
>
> Wilfred Owen, 'Strange Meeting'

It was early 1942, and Dad was sixteen. At his parents' request, the Perse School put him through a test to determine what he should do with his life.

'He is a boy of very good ability,' the assessor opined. 'Our suggestions in approximate order of suitability are perhaps, first, a preliminary degree in estate management at London University. Second, perhaps a degree in economics at London University, with a view to becoming a statistician, a factory inspector, or an accountant. The decision between these three need not be made until nearer the end of his degree course. Third, a degree in engineering with a view to becoming a factory inspector. Fourth, accountancy, serving articled clerkship of five years, without a preliminary degree. Or fifth, aeronautical or electrical engineering.' I half expected a sixth alternative: 'Perhaps a PhD in nuclear physics, with a view to becoming a factory inspector.'

The author seemed to be advertising London University, and the dad I had would have been stupefied by most of these options. Regardless, the world was in flames. I know what would have happened had I been eighteen in 1914 or 1939: I would have rushed off to get killed, no questions asked. Albert was not keen on his teenage son signing up to go to war. Dad went to his mother, since no matter what arguments she might put up, he would prevail. Sure enough, she helped him fake his date of birth and get into the RAF. He was colour-blind, so they would not let him be a pilot; the RAF careers adviser told him to become a navigator. In 1943, he headed off to Port Elizabeth in South Africa for his basic training, and by the next year he found himself in Italy, just like his father twenty-seven years earlier.

Dad was with Bomber Command. He may have been young and keen to play his part, but he was soon aghast at the reality of raining bombs down on people he had never met. He transferred to the Pathfinders, who would go ahead and drop flares over the target. He rationalised that fewer innocent people would be killed if his navigation was accurate. The mortality rate of Pathfinders was high, sometimes due to the flak and sometimes to the strain in the cockpit. Dad didn't talk about it often but he told one story: His Lancaster was traversing the Alps back from a target in Germany, and both pilots, exhausted from the missions and from living life on fast-forward, fuelled by amphetamines, had drifted off to sleep. Dad sensed that something was wrong, and as he looked up from his maps he saw they were headed towards a mountain. He woke them just in time.

Auntie Jean later speculated that perhaps the stress of his RAF service might have tipped Dad over the edge. Why would it not? Dad was in Rome, still only nineteen years old, on VE Day. As with Albert before him, it was time to come home.

My parents met at the Newmarket golf course in 1946. The fairway was an important venue for the youthful middle class, and the nineteenth hole was their social epicentre. My mother was Jean Thomas, and confusingly she had begun to play with Dad's sister Jean. (The next seventy years would be a confusion of Jeans. I shall refer to my mother as Mum, since that is what I have always called her.)

It is difficult to assess one's parents objectively, and I think for many years I underestimated Mum. She was, like Dad's sister, an intelligent and adventurous woman who was limited by the accidental era of her birth. Auntie Jean had been disappointed in 'her war', as she had been working as a secretary for the British Aluminium Company and had wanted to do more, like her gallant young brother in the RAF. My mother was younger, but had similar aspirations.

Mum had found love for the first time in 1931, when she was nearly five, and it blossomed in her own mind for a decade. 'My first love affair came to an abrupt end when I was fourteen,' she told me once, 'but it was a beautiful experience and made its impression upon me for the rest of my life.' She thought herself an unattractive child, with a crop of freckles and owl-like spectacles which gave her a curious dignity, topped by unmanageable ginger hair. Jim London, on the other hand, was any young girl's dream. 'Brown-skinned, slim, with an attractive, impish face and an altogether engaging character,' she remembered. 'He was my distant cousin, and my pretty elder sister Ann and I spent every summer holiday with him and his sister at their Cornish seaside home.'

I did not understand Mum's hang-up about her sister. Looking at pictures from back then, they were clearly sisters, and I would no more describe Ann as pretty than I would say Mum was not. Jim, on the other hand, was rakish. 'He was always the one who led the way into the darkest caves, who thought up the most daredevil escapades, who caught the most shrimps, and who, if we built a monster sandcastle, would stand on his head on top of it,' Mum recalled. 'But he always took me along – an unprepossessing child – while his older, vivacious sister and Ann conspired about weightier matters more suited to their superior age.'

Mum also wondered why Jim was so good to her. I suspect it is because she underrated herself and was, in many ways, more interesting to talk to than other girls. 'In between these holidays we would write long letters to each other – I always did enjoy writing letters, and it was certainly worth it for the joy of getting one of Jim's in return.' He joined the Merchant Navy, and the last time Mum saw him was Sunday, 3 September 1939, the day Britain declared war. He later sent her a glamorous photograph of himself wearing the uniform of a midshipman in Malta, on Christmas Day 1940, just before the Stukas dive-bombed his ship, the M V *Essex*. The target was the aircraft carrier H M S *Illustrious*, but *Essex* was docked beside her.

Later, when she took her exams at the age of fifteen and a half, Mum scored her top mark in Written French. She resolved, with a friend, that this was her call to arms. The two of them took a train to London, walked to King Charles Street in Whitehall, and announced themselves ready to parachute into France to join La Résistance. On our trips to the Continent when I was growing up Mum knew all the words, but she sounded even more British than Colonel Horden, who taught me prep-school French in the tones of a parade-ground officer of the Raj. I had an image of her writing out her replies to the German officer in any interrogation, to disguise her awful accent. Fortunately it did not come to that, as a nice young chap in the Foreign Office gave them tea and said to come back when they were eighteen – which, it transpired, was too late.

Rejected for active duty, Mum was forced down a more traditional path and did a secretarial course in London. Seventy years later, I was trying to work out how to get British people to empathise with the people of Waziristan, in Pakistan's tribal region. They were being terrorised by Predator drones hurling Hellfire missiles at them. I asked Mum about her experiences in the Blitz and her mind's eye went immediately back to Sunday, 18 June 1944. She had decided to go into her secretarial school on Buckingham Palace Road to get some work done, and a doodlebug hit the Guards' Chapel, killing 121 people and shattering the windows of her office. She described it vividly – even though by that stage in life her recent memories were fading.

23

Everyone was glad that the peace had come. Mum began to develop a relationship with Dad, who returned to Cambridge on a grant for ex-servicemen to read for a degree in estate management – just as his careers adviser had suggested, though thankfully the university had no degree option in Factory Inspection. As a former Pathfinder he was allowed to take his degree in two years instead of three, and he worked hard, getting a first. But even if the war had slightly loosened the shackles of class, the university gave Dad a sense of inferiority. Indeed, rather than be plain Dick Smith, he started using his middle name, Stafford, giving himself a double-barrelled surname. When he formally changed it, he did not pay the extra couple of pounds to add a hyphen.

By the mid-1950s, my parents had been 'dating' for seven years. Mum was twenty-nine, and her sister already had a family in faraway New Zealand. Mum had waited long enough. On 9 May 1955, they were coming from a game of golf in Cambridge, with Dad driving her green Morris 8. She told him it was time to put up or shut up. He immediately swerved to the side of the road and proposed to her. They married two months later in Fordham Parish Church, exiting into the sunshine with crossed golf clubs held above them.

'So where exactly did he propose to you? I want the full romantic story,' I insisted.

'Hmm.' We were talking many years later, long after the divorce, and she lacked nostalgia, so it was not easy to pull it out of her. She thought back. 'When he pulled the car over . . . it was past Station Road before you get to the bridge, not too far from Addenbrooke's Hospital. Right across from Fulbourn Asylum.'

That was where Great-Granny Frances had been sectioned.

'I suppose it might have told me something . . .' Mum said.

3

Larry Lonchar's Destiny: The Electric Chair

So many times in my life I went left when I should have gone right, and I went right when I should have gone left. It was mistake after mistake after mistake.

Last words of death row prisoner Robert Towery (1991).

When I first came to know Larry Lonchar, in 1986, he was thirty-five years old, and though he had once been six feet tall, he was already shrinking. The tide of his thin blond hair was almost completely out. His walk was more a shuffle, and if you had followed his footprints along a sandy beach, you would have noticed that they splayed like a duck's. While Larry loved sports of any sort on the yard, any success was due more to determination than athleticism.

Above the belt, Larry was developing the slight protuberance of creeping middle age. When he pulled up the leg of his uniform trousers, I noticed that he had virtually no hair. That is the kind of detail that is, perversely, highlighted when you sit with a death row client in Georgia, a state that clung vengefully to the electric chair until 2001. The executioner would be grateful that there was so little to shave off the right shin to make a good contact.

Sometimes, in summer, when Larry would go without an undershirt, wisps of blond hair would peep out from his chest. This did not happen often, though, for he was particular about his appearance. He always wore the right amount of inexpensive cologne, and he would refuse a visit if the guards had not allowed him sufficient time to shower and shave. I was annoyed when he first did this to me. After all, wasn't I the busy lawyer who had driven miles to see him? Later, I realised that Larry was trying to preserve that simple dignity. He did not live in an English village, and I could not arrive unannounced for a spot of tea.

Larry had come a long way from Michigan to his small home in Cell Block G, at the euphemistically named Georgia Diagnostic and Classification Center – death row.

Larry's family had emigrated from Yugoslavia. His grandmother Victoria was thirteen years old when she arrived on a boat in 1928. Paying for the rite of passage across the Atlantic was the goal of many Great War–weary Europeans. Larry's grandfather Milan Lonchar Sr had come to America earlier, but returned to his native country and bought the rights to Victoria. He met her off the boat, taking her to his new home in Chicago. Under the terms of her dowry, she soon began bearing him children.

These were the Prohibition years. Naturally, since alcohol was banned by constitutional amendment, human nature dictated that more liquor be consumed per person than at any time before or since. Milan Sr opened some lucrative speakeasies on the streets of Eliot Ness and Al Capone. When he drank, he beat his wife. This was one of the immutable laws of Lonchar nature.

Larry's father, Milan Jr, was four when Victoria ran away to Battle Creek, Michigan. The town had long been headquarters to Kellogg's corn flakes. Now it became home to the Lonchars. She never saw her husband again.

'The family only heard tell of Milan Sr once more,' said Larry. 'When my father was sixteen, seventeen years old, word came in Battle Creek that my grandfather had died and my grandmother was to get all of her husband's inheritance. She coulda had a fortune, Grandma, but she didn't want no part of it.' Larry seemed proud that his grandmother had taken a stand.

But, however righteous, her decision was a sore that itched the family. When Milan Jr was old enough for his turn at getting drunk, he would beat his own mother for depriving him of his birthright. Usually, he would hold her by the hair and smack her in the face again and again with his balled-up fist. He would be crying all the time as he did it. 'Because of you I'll never have nothing,' he would wail between blows.

Alone in Battle Creek with her children in the 1930s, her situation as depressed as the country's, Victoria met and married another alcoholic and abusive Yugoslav, Dan Dibjak. Larry would come to know Dan as his grandfather.

Larry's mother, Elsie Lick, was seventeen when she met Milan Jr in June 1947, shortly after my own mother first encountered my father on the Newmarket golf course. 'We met on a dark and rainy Friday the 13th . . . I guess I should have taken that for the sign that it was,' Elsie recalled sadly, echoing my mother's sardonic comment about Dad's proposal.

Like many in Battle Creek, Elsie and Milan Jr were both working their first jobs in the packing department of the Kellogg's cereal factory. They married on Valentine's Day 1948. Their first son was given the name Milan (the third), but Grandmother Victoria soon nicknamed him Chooch. The house shook every time a train went by, and his sobriquet came from the first word he spoke.

The rheumatic Chooch was premature. The doctors blamed it on the turpentine poisoning that a pregnant Elsie suffered when in a closed room stripping furniture for their new home. Chooch then contracted polio, the fearsome disease that had put Franklin D. Roosevelt in a wheelchair. He spent the first year of his life in the hospital.

The second child – Paul 'Tiny' Lonchar – came home before his older brother. Nobody could really remember why he was called Tiny. He was neither particularly big nor small. The most memorable part of him by the time I knew him was his thick black moustache, surrounded by his rather pockmarked cheeks. As a child, he took the sickly Chooch to school as a 'show and tell' exhibit. There he explained to his classmates that Chooch had never been well enough to attend school himself.

Larry, the third child, arrived on 3 September 1951. He was followed by Christina (Chris) and John.

Larry's father quit his job with Kellogg's to work as a brakeman on the Grand Trunk Railroad, where he plied the Battle Creek–Chicago line. Railroad life fertilised his alcoholic gene: in the local community, the service was known as the Grand Trunk Drunk Line.

'Although my mother started drinking later, I'd say by the time she reached full capacity, the two of them were pretty much neck and neck in the amount of liquor they drank,' Chris remembered with a blend of sadness and anger. 'They'd both put away a bottle of vodka a day. When we'd come home from school, we'd find her passed out on the kitchen table. If she was lucky, she'd've made it to the bedroom floor. Us kids never could bring anyone home, 'cause we'd never know what we'd find there.'

Chooch's medical problems, combined with the parents' addictions, placed an immense strain on the family in a country with little welfare and no national health service. 'Mom was sick a lot with "nerves" and anything else you could think of,' Tiny recalled. 'She'd take any pills, even Chooch's, because she believed in popping things. She used to say they made her forget what the doctors told her she needed to forget.'

'Nerves' was a common euphemism. Elsie built up her medical stocks, and eventually clothes were displaced by pills in four dresser drawers. She would mix and match so often that she barely left the house, and then generally only to visit the local tavern. The Lonchar children were alone most of the time.

When my own father somehow got out of his parents' sight and was hit by a car, he was five. Larry was rather younger.

Tiny was sitting on the kerb when his little brother, still a toddler, wandered into the street and sat down to play. A car did not notice him until too late. 'It ran right over him,' Tiny said. 'It tried to stop, but by the time the tyres finished squealing, Larry was already underneath. They backed up again, and caught his head on the front bumper a second time.'

In a country with proper medical care, he would have been taken to the emergency room. Instead Larry's father came home, picked him up and put him to bed. As the family relates it, Larry 'slept for a long time'. Like my father, he was unconscious, probably in a coma. Had there been an ambulance for the lawyers to chase, the accident could have been worth millions. But for Larry, it was only worth a head injury – perhaps another qualification for his death row destiny. When I sat with him in the visiting room in Georgia, Larry would periodically stare into the distance. He would seem oblivious of whatever was said to him, and his eyes would bulge before rolling up under his lids. I wondered whether I was witnessing the sequelae of the accident.

Larry injured himself in other ways as he grew up. 'He was never too good at judging spaces or distances,' Tiny recalled. Truth be told, Larry was not too good at judging anything. 'Larry was playing catcher in Little League softball when he was about eight. He got too close to the batter, who was looking for a home run. Instead, he caught Larry right around the head. Knocked him stone cold. Like always, we took him home and put him to bed. I don't think my folks was even 'round that day, and weren't none of us kids thinking about hospital.'

Chris smiled when she described her brother. 'Larry was the kind of kid who would take a step at the corner, and when he'd turn, he'd walk right into the wall and bash his head.' Meanwhile, the family's finances were strained to the point that the barkeeper refused further credit, and they moved in with the grandparents, Dan and Victoria, on Stone Avenue. There the five children shared beds in the stone basement, with its cement floor. Michigan is on the Great Lakes, and winter smothers the state with snow for several months. Going to the loo in the night meant going upstairs. There were any number of situations to find up there: Elsie might be passed out, and Milan gone to Chicago or the tavern; Milan might be coming home drunk to wake Elsie up and beat her; Milan might catch sight of the kids and beat them instead.

'When the drink would catch a hold of Dad, and Dad would catch a hold of you, that's when he'd grab you by the shoulder or a bunch of hair, and he'd hold you real tight,' Larry told me, staring up at the ceiling of the visiting room and sighing deeply. I needed to know about his background, to put together some kind of a case for him, but he hated to talk about it. Larry hated snitches above all else in life, and talking trash about the family was like snitching. Still, sometimes he would open up without any warning. It seemed as if the pain of his childhood had forced its way to the surface just long enough for him to be angry.

'Dad'd already have rolled up his belt around the other hand, with the buckle hanging out the end. Then he'd swing. He'd be drunk, and your aim gets messed up when you're drunk, so I don't guess he'd be trying to hit any one part of you. Just any-where on you . . .' He continued staring at the ceiling. 'Don't guess it was funny, but it must've looked pretty funny. You'd be squirming and kicking out like an Indian, and he'd be after you with that buckle. You'd be trying to get away, 'cause you knew this wasn't like you'd get your ten licks now or your ten licks later. I mean . . . Dad used to ask us where all those welts and sores on our bodies come from. No, no . . . if you got away that's usually all you had to do. Wait till he passed out. He never remembered he was mad in the morning.'

All in all, he said, the smart move was to stay in the damp basement. 'Sure, if Mom or Dad was home we'd stay in the basement most of the time,' Tiny agreed. 'But a big, loud fight between the two of them usually got at least me and Larry out to make sure my father didn't kill my mother. I'd say maybe once a week. When he was drunk, I think sometimes he wanted to kill her. He'd be holding her hair, beating her. But I kinda understand what he was going through. Sometimes, we all wanted to kill her.' Tiny paused then, momentarily back in the basement of his childhood. We were talking on a steaming Georgia afternoon, yet I watched his moustache twitch as he shivered. 'She was supposed to be our mother. But you'd come home from school and find her passed out on the floor. Or she'd cry, and tell us she was sick, and ask us for money for more booze. And here we were, nine, ten years old. Chris and Larry, they'd give her their pocket money.'

The parents began to match each other in affairs as well as vodka. 'Mom, she'd bring the neighbour Ray down to the basement, so that he could get out if they heard my dad coming in from the bar,' Larry told me, staring up at the ceiling again. 'Of course, that was our bedroom. So I was there, hiding behind the sheets. There was all this noise, gruntin' an' all. She must've been real drunk. I called out to her. But she never said a word to me. Not once.'

The affair with Ray was whispered about around town. One night their father poured extra alcohol onto the smouldering hearth of his resentment. 'We heard the two of them go at it upstairs again. I remember thinking it was a little early for them to be so heavy into fighting,' Tiny said. 'It was winter in that basement, but I was trying on some new swimming trunks I'd been given, and I wasn't wearing nothing else when I peeked through the door at the top of the stairs. Couldn't do nothing but stand there and scream ourselves. My mother was in her bathrobe. He must've picked her out of bed. Her feet was bare. My father was holding her by the shoulders real hard. Her face was already messed up. He had on these big boots and he was stomping her feet with his heels. He was screaming over and over and over again, "See if you ever run around on me again! See if you ever run around on me again! See if you ever run around on me again!" He'd say that every stomp. Then he drug her out into the snow. I'll never forget that snow. I still only had my trunks on. Don't know, but it felt like he beat her out there for thirty whole minutes. Larry stayed out there when I finally went in to call the *po*-lice.'

This was not the first time they had dialled the emergency number. Every now and then, when Milan failed to pass out early in the evening, one of the children had called them. It never amounted to much. Then, even more than now, the police believed that domestic disharmony was not a matter requiring outside intervention. None of the family had any respect for the *po*-lice.

'They arrived too late again,' Tiny went on. 'By that time, my father'd got her inside the screen door. Just told the cops everything was fine, and they went on and left . . . pretty much what they always did. But after they left, he come after me 'n' Larry next. We called the police again, but by the time they got there he'd passed out in his chair.'

Tiny and Larry had escaped, but Elsie had long-term physical damage. 'My mother's feet, they've tried to get them to do right, but they don't any more.'

Not long after, Milan decided that it was his turn to desert the family. Elsie ought to have been glad, but she had grown psychologically dependent on the cycle of violence. Now her life seemed to be finished. She vacillated between the certainty that one of the neighbours was trying to kill her, and loud pronouncements that she was going to kill herself. As Larry entered the muddled years of his adolescence, she told him daily that someone was going to take his life. Gradually, she became more prescient, and insisted that his assassins would be the *po*-lice.

Sure enough, he was soon in trouble with the authorities. Larry had done well in his early classroom years. His best subject was arithmetic. 'Then,' reported one of his many probation officers, 'very suddenly, our defendant began to have serious problems.' Larry's arrests became more frequent. This gave

Elsie more cause to blame her 'nerves' on him. She saw the strange eye movements, followed by unexplained fits of rage.

'I saw Larry's eyes walling back in his head,' Elsie remembered when I quizzed her on Larry's youth. 'Nothing but the whites of his eyes remained.' Her voice was as vacant as her own eyes; the cigarette rasp had been softened by encroaching emphysema. Her blonde hair had seen years of corrosive bleach. 'One time, Larry hit me during one of his tantrums,' she went on reluctantly. She, too, felt she was betraying her son by revealing important truths. 'A few days later I brought it up with him, and he acted like I was joking. I could hardly convince him that he had done it.'

Some minor infraction prompted Miss White, his maths teacher, to order Larry to leave the classroom. 'You ol' bitch!' he yelled at her. For this heinous offence he was sent to a juvenile court and adjudicated a delinquent. With his mother's complicity, he was committed to the Marshall Juvenile Delinquent Home. This was sufficiently far away to provide Elsie with an excuse not to visit her son. 'I don't know how long he stayed there, or anything about his life there,' she said. 'When he got out, Milan and I were divorcing, and I was in the middle of a nervous breakdown. When he came home, I went to the sanatorium.'

Elsie's hangovers had warped into psychosis. She had no health insurance for proper treatment and the hospital found it convenient to place her in four-point restraints, strapping her down by the wrists and ankles. Perhaps it was not so different to my great-grandmother Frances's experience in her paupers' asylum half a century before. When Larry got out of his own institution, he visited his mother. Elsie screamed for him to wipe off the crawling bugs and blow on her burning feet.

Larry could never accept his parents' split. He had internalised his mother's constant complaints, and blamed himself for the break-up. One of the first faceless psychologists who evaluated Larry recorded that he was 'plagued with feelings of insecurity and inadequacy which are grossly disproportionate to his realistic situation'. Everything was his fault. Gradually, Larry came to inherit his mother's fascination with death. This acorn later grew into his oak tree of obsession: the only way he could ever stop causing his family problems would be to volunteer for the electric chair.

When she got out of the hospital, Elsie was on the limited welfare that America provides. Milan had been ordered to find $50 in child support – just $10 per child per week. True to the Lonchar family tradition, he would not pay even this paltry sum. Elsie lived off her disability cheque. To support her five children and her various drug dependencies, she received $2,520 a year.

Most of the children planned their escape from an early age. Larry was the one who could not stand to leave his mother alone. He was scared for her. But he kept exchanging home for a prison cell. He was seventeen when he went to the Battle Creek County Jail on an adult prosecution; then he injured an officer, Howard McPharlin, during an escape, and picked up another charge, though McPharlin told me he liked Larry when I called him many years later.

'I do believe that deep inside,' Elsie said, 'Larry was scared to live at home, so he would do things to be sent back to institutions every time he got out.' As I went through his old records, I found that he was just twenty when the psychologists came to the same diagnosis: Larry felt that prison was the only safe place for him, where he could fit in without seeing himself as a source of pain for his family.

Dr M. J. Keyser was a clinical psychologist performing routine evaluations at the reception centre for the Michigan Department of Corrections. His report rolled off a typewriter with a smudged ribbon. Larry got on so well 'in the institutional setting that his difficulties have been ignored to the point where he finds greater rewards in committing antisocial acts and achieving a return to the institution. He almost impulsively got into trouble.'

In 1978, another state expert asked Larry why he kept coming back. At the time he had a job (albeit a McJob). He was waiting for some college grades (though a degree might lead him into some McDebt). Despite this, Larry held up a store. He was polite, and nobody was hurt. He was soon caught. 'I don't know why I do this shit,' Larry said to the psychologist. 'I guess . . . what've I got to lose? You guys got me institutionalised. I ask you not to send me right back out there, and you do. I don't know how to make it on my own out there. Now they just send me back to prison and I think of that as my home.'

'It is obvious to this agent,' said probation officer Timothy G. McCaleb, 'that Mr Lonchar is, through the mechanism of well-planned and "politely executed" armed robberies, forcing the criminal justice system to become an accomplice in his own destruction. He seems driven to these acts by an overwhelming conviction that he cannot make it on the outside, along with a pervasive feeling of self-disgust, and the resulting incarceration and punishment deals with both of those feelings.'

At least the Michigan Department of Corrections did not bother you if you did not bother them. The inmates ran the institution, and Larry knew that there was far more honour among thieves than in the outside world. Nobody stole from his pale green prison chest. His normally nervous eyes were inscrutable when he was bluffing in a game of poker. But the paradox of his hopelessness was that he could not even succeed at failing. The prison officers liked him so much, and he adapted himself so well, that he was always recommended for early parole. He would then be ushered out of the prison gate, his old leather suitcase holding nothing but the suit he had worn to court four years before. He had only one life plan: getting back in without hurting anyone.

4

Fractures in Paradise:
The Manic-Depressive Temperament

Rough winds do shake the darling buds of May
And summer's lease hath all too short a date.

William Shakespeare, Sonnet 18

I arrived on my parents' fourth wedding anniversary, 9 July 1959. My older siblings, Mark and Mary, had been born in 1957 and 1958. I had to have a blood transfusion to make it through my first few days. Yet I was born into privilege. Dad was working in the Department of Estate Management at Cambridge, and had just inherited the oldest stud farm in the world.

Cheveley Park was an extraordinary place to grow up. Our home, Garden House, was set at the end of a long drive, shaded by the Domesday Book cedar trees. There was a large open garage to the right, with a ten-foot brick wall that ran thirty yards to the glass front entrance. The garage had a rear exit leading to the run that belonged to Vesta (the goddess of the hearth), our black Labrador. Beyond was the tennis court and the dark woodsheds where the chickens used to brood and Mary once tempted me to try a cigarette when I was five years old. A beech wood ran away along the fence where once the horses of royalty had thundered towards the finish line of the old racetrack. The start of each year was marked by an army of snowdrops among the roots, surrounded by the aconites and the crocuses, before the yellow daffodils pushed through.

On the west side of the house the lawn spread out in front of my bedroom window – past the ancient apple tree to a row of fuchsias. It was a tranquil space, enclosed by another ten-foot brick wall. One right quarter was partitioned into squares of gooseberry bushes, with a dovecote above them. The red-painted door in the far left corner let out into another large walled area with two ranks of greenhouses in an L-shape, a hundred yards in one direction, fifty in the other. Everything that grew here was for home consumption, and as a child I would walk through, inhaling the smouldering scent of a hundred tomato plants.

Behind the garden was a row of hazel and yew trees, where my friend Anthony and I used to cut bows and arrows to hunt imaginary Norman sheriffs around the three hundred acres of the estate. Anthony was the youngest son of Peter Rossdale, the famous equine vet; we were born within weeks of each other and remained inseparable for the first eight years of our lives. We built castles out of bales in the barns until the stud groom, Bill Cowell, chased us away with his booming retired-sergeant-major voice and, as often as not, a false threat with his shotgun.

While it was all beyond me at this point, the stud was doing well. On 11 September 1961, my mother noted that it was mortgage-free for the first time since Albert's death, when death duties had been imposed. Psidium was the leading stallion standing at stud. That June he had won the Derby as a 66-1 outsider in 2 minutes, 36.4 seconds, going away from the field. I looked him up against all the other winners since 1780: he was seven seconds quicker than the famous Isinglass had been in 1893.

The same year, my mother spent a £3,000 bequest from her aunt on No. 5, The Crescent, in Cromer, largely because that had been Dad's seaside resort when he was a child, full of fond memories. It was a fantastical, sea-air-decayed, four-storey holiday home overlooking the slipway. We would go there in the winter months as well, pouring coins into the electricity meter to start the heating, and I would sit on the cushioned window ledge with rain lashing the glass, as the waves crashed on the beach far below. There I would watch the ships inching along the grey horizon.

In Cromer, Dad would be the perfect father. He sat on the beach, on a red-and-white camping chair, staring contemplatively out to sea with his pipe. Here his passions were the Cromer crabs and the kippers selected carefully from Mr Davies's shoebox-size shop. Sometimes, when we heard the rusting tractors backfiring into life in the early morning, preparing to haul the boats in, Dad would take one of us to go and negotiate for fresh mackerel. Later in the day we might head to Blakeney Point, where we would spend the afternoon stooping for cockles and mussels, which would then soak in the bath, pitting the enamel.

The most exciting moments were down on the esplanade in a winter gale, when Mary and I would duck behind the massive concrete wall as the waves crashed over. Sometimes the siren would call the lifeboatmen to their task, and we would watch the unsinkable craft slide down the slipway at the end of the pier, colliding with the North Sea in a spray. For years we had a tall brown Henry Blogg mug, commemorating the most famous of the RNLI coxswains.

Dad would sometimes overdo his bonhomie and could be an astoundingly reckless driver. He had a Triumph Vitesse, and one time, when I was travelling up to Cromer with him alone, he announced that in the seventy-five miles we were going to overtake one hundred other cars. We overtook the hundredth vehicle, dangerously, by going at twice the speed limit just as we came into the town. It seemed to me that Dad would never fail when he set himself a challenge.

Back at the stud, Mark was generally closeted in his room, reading a book a day – from an early age, he rationed himself to one science-fiction novel for every two works of non-fiction. He would periodically emerge with his metal detector, searching for the coins of the wealthy punters on what had once been the stands of the Cheveley Park racecourse, now thick with brambles. Or he would get in his ancient black van with a square hole cut in the roof, and position his polished brass telescope to study the stars at night.

Mary had her pony in its walled paddock. I didn't like riding; she tried to encourage me when I was just four by slapping the pony. I hung on for a few steps, before subsiding down the side of the animal into a fresh pile of manure.

If the setting was bucolic, my experience of family was idyllic. Dad ran the stud, and Mum worked in the snug office between the hall and the lounge. Ivy Phillips, the secretary, typed away there too, and after her husband died she used to come over most evenings and read to me. There were only two characters I would countenance, Robin Hood and Brer Rabbit. My bedroom was off the long, carpeted landing, next to Mary's. The headboard of my bed was hard against a joist that ran up to the ceiling. Periodically, a mouse would run along it. Some in the household wanted him dealt with, but I would let nobody persecute my friend. There was also a velvety green, tasselled bedspread, ridged like a perfectly ploughed field – its colour consistent with my dreams of Sherwood Forest.

Dad would occasionally put me to bed, always reciting poetry. He had a resonant voice and he would lean back at the foot of the bed, close his eyes and quote away, perhaps 'Ozymandias' by Shelley, or Rossetti's 'Up-hill'. I absorbed his favourites by osmosis. I have a strong sense of Dad's smell, which I associate with what a father should be. His jacket gave off male sweat – a fatherly smell, it seemed to me at the time – and I can still feel the rough five o'clock shadow of his cheek from the few times my skin touched his. He used an electric shaver in the morning in my parents' bathroom, craning his neck up as he caught the more difficult parts, sometimes talking to me as he did it.

The stud came with a crew of twenty-three who were invariably kind to us as kids. There were the two gardeners, who turned a blind eye to the larceny of their tomatoes. Alf Ottley, the carpenter, let us swipe the sponge cake his wife Beryl had put in for his tea. Dad seemed to be in his element on the stud. He would be leaning on the fence, pipe in hand, discussing the foals with Mr Cowell, or with Fred Baker and Jimmy Allington, the stallion men. He would scoop Mary up to nuzzle a favourite mare. He would explain how the ivy was killing off the avenue of beech trees near the main entrance, and pay us one shilling an hour to cut it back. He would get us up early to go rooting around for fresh mushrooms in the paddock near Gypsy Walk, bringing them back so Mum could fry them with kidneys for breakfast.

Every Sunday there was the trip down Duchess Drive to All Saints Church in Newmarket, where we would listen to Reverend Tony Winter, followed by a formal lunch. This was a mildly trying experience for a young lad. I blamed the Church of England for the fact that I had to wear National Health Service glasses from the age of five, as I was hauled to the optician after I could not make out the hymn numbers. The word of God was generally of no interest to my wandering young mind, and the ensuing Sunday meal at Winston Churchill's dining-room table rivalled the earlier sermon for interminability.

Only once do I remember wanting to stay at lunch. Two Jehovah's Witnesses happened upon our glass front door around noon on a Sunday, and Dad half hauled them in for lunch, commanding us to lay two extra places at the table. He then verbally assaulted them over their interpretation of the Bible for two hours, starting with a minor skirmish over sherry in the lounge and culminating in the *coup de grâce* over apple crumble and custard. At the time, I thought it was Dad at his very finest, dissecting them as he sharpened the carving knife.

Dad relished it when someone took an alternative perspective to life. One evening, Mum invited him to mediate a debate I was having with her about whether I could stay up to see more of the dreadful television my older siblings were watching. He demanded of me whether I preferred to go to bed late and get up late, or go to bed early and get up early. I said I preferred to go to bed late and get up early. I dare say I was only trying to get my own way, but Dad was thrilled that I was fighting his hypothetical. He ruled in my favour.

I was a very shy child, seen in photographs grasping my mother's skirt, half hidden. I soon could hide no more. By the age of seven I was over five feet tall, always the biggest in my class, and my nickname was Dustbin as I would eat anything in sight.

We went skiing each winter. Every now and then Dad would again go too far. En route to Austria, he was driving with Mary in his latest Triumph when he hit black ice at speed, and spun the car over the lip of the road into a snow-covered field. With no roll bar, and a soft roof, it was a miracle that they both emerged unscathed. Later on that holiday we were in a music hall, on a balcony over the main floor, watching the men in lederhosen slap their thighs and squeeze their accordions. Someone along from us accidentally knocked a glass over and it fell onto the table below, provoking a number of blond Aryan youths to rush up the stairs for revenge. Mum shepherded us out, but Dad stayed behind to get into an uncomprehending argument with some drunks who did not speak English. He had been a boxer at Cambridge, and with the war only twenty years past, he was not going to walk away from a bunch of Austrians. He came back to the apartment with a shiner of an eye. Mum took a slab of meat out of the fridge to calm the swelling, while I looked on, already composing the dramatic – fictional – essay I would write when I got back to school, about my own role in the adventure.

Even in winter, there was little reason to think that this eternal summer would ever come to an end. Dad had *joie de vivre* and did not want to let a day go by without marvelling at the tableau of creation. As we motored along, singing 'It's a Long Way to Tipperary', he might swerve into a lay-by at any moment and force us out of the car to admire a view of the Rhine or the towering Alps. His favourite word was 'enthusiasm'. He would bang on about this all the time, and say it came from the Greek and meant 'imbued with God'.

I cannot imagine many parents want their children deeply involved in politics before primary school begins, but Dad did. He would obsess about the injustices that were perpetrated against others. He encouraged my brother to start a correspondence with the Shah of Iran about population control. He read books very rarely, but when something caught his imagination, he got carried away. When he was given a history of the Irish potato famine, he made me, aged six, read parts of it, to understand the horrors that the English absentee landlords had inflicted.

So, for the first few years of my life, the sea seemed calm and deep blue. But long before I had any sense of it, the waters were roiling underneath the surface.

In the early sixties, Dad was working two jobs. He had stayed on with the Department of Estate Management at Cambridge, charged with planning the investments of various colleges. At the same time, he was meant to be running the stud.

I had no idea at the time, but he had a breakdown in 1963. The cine film of 9 July captures Chelsea Pensioners at my fourth birthday party in the garden. Dad had paid for them all to come up by coach from London for the day to look around the stud. Two dozen grizzled old guys who had fought in the Great War, in scarlet uniforms with ranks of medals, were kicking my football into the fuchsias. They left me a painted plaster of Paris Pensioner who stood guard at my bedside for years afterwards.

Around the beginning of that September, as I started at Fairstead House Primary School, Dad tried to commit the university to £40,000 of unauthorised expenditure on a development in Cambridge, because he decided he knew best and the fuddy-duddies had been too slow in acting. The university was horrified (it was a million pounds in today's money) and came down hard on him.

'After that incident, he was in a deep depression,' my mother told me years later. 'He was suffering from insomnia. He could make no decisions, he thought everything was going wrong.' Dad was sectioned in Kent for some weeks, near his sister, to avoid Newmarket people knowing. As far as anyone was concerned, he was recuperating from illness; the university gave him time off on medical grounds, saying he had been overworking. I had no idea anything had happened. Dad had simply gone away for a bit.

This was the first and only time that Dad accepted treatment. His primary physician was a psychiatrist of renown, Dr Richard Hunter. Hunter's mother, Ida Wertheimer, was German and Jewish. She was also a psychiatrist. When Adolf Hitler became Chancellor on 30 January 1933, she left Berlin and took her two children to London.

Hunter dissented from many of the sacred cows of his profession. He felt that there was a tendency to seize on a medication that seemed to impact the symptoms of a disorder without understanding its aetiology. This reflected the worst of medicine from preceding centuries. He gave the example of bleeding: once, a physician's solution to everything had been to 'rebalance' the humours in the body. Perhaps a physician tried bloodletting and saw that it had a beneficial effect on hypertension, temporarily reducing blood pressure. Without understanding the connection, an entire pseudoscience arose out of this one observation, and soon a British medical text recommended bloodletting as a cure for everything from acne to asthma.

The brain, Hunter thought, was a physical organism, while the notion of a 'mind' was mostly a confabulation created by humans to make themselves feel better (akin to inventing heaven or an afterlife). The psychiatric profession would see an 'emotional' disorder where advances in medicine were gradually revealing a physiological or neurological explanation.

★

I have sympathy with Hunter's views. Many years later, in 1990, I took on the case of Troy Dugar, a fifteen-year-old kid on death row in Louisiana, and schizophrenia became the focal point of a case for the first time in my then-nascent career. I could certainly see the manifestations of illness – Troy would lie handcuffed to the bed in the Louisiana State Prison hospital, picking imaginary insects off his arms, just as Elsie Lonchar had done. Later, when we were in court together, his ankles shackled to the floor, he started giggling.

I leaned over and whispered. 'What's up, Troy?'

He turned to me, his eyes glittering. We were in the old Calcasieu Parish Courthouse, where oak panelling lined the high walls. He indicated above the bench where Judge Arthur Planchard was seated, staring at us disapprovingly through thick glasses. 'The judge!' he exclaimed in a stage whisper, clearly audible, echoing about us. 'He's floating up . . . he's drooling all down the side of his mouth!' His voice rose in manic joy. The judge frowned some more.

I became obsessed with trying to understand Troy's illness. He was being forced to take haloperidol, an early and cheap antipsychotic much used in prison. He hated the medicine. I read about tardive dyskinesia, the palsied spasms that came as a side effect. The more I read, the more appalled I was: according to a learned account of this process, 'the history of antipsychotic drug development has had a long and torturous course, often based on chance findings that bear little relationship to the intellectual background driving observations'. As early as 1891 the drug was being used for malaria. By chance, six decades later, in the 1950s, when a person suffering from schizophrenia also contracted malaria, doctors noticed that it seemingly helped temper his psychosis. Over the next twenty years, some forty such antipsychotic drugs were introduced to the world. Obviously the drugs were treating something physiological, but nobody was sure how they worked. They were effectively experimenting on humans.

As I delved more into the literature on schizophrenia, I came across tentative research indicating a genetic predisposition to the illness. There was plenty of similar work on bipolar disorder, and if there is a genetic predisposition, it almost certainly means that those of us who are more likely to suffer from it have a particular, perhaps mutant, gene. In other words, that which we deem 'mental' is actually in large part 'physiological' – if there is really a sensible distinction between the two. An external event might trigger something – such as the shocking impact Dad and Larry experienced when they were each run over by a car, or the stress placed on Dad when he was required to bomb Germany while still a teenager – but both had inherited a particular gene.

This was Dr Hunter's view. Dad would have liked Hunter's general attitude, as the man questioned the authorities of his profession. Unfortunately, though, Dad did not like Hunter's conclusion: Stafford Smith, he opined, did exhibit the symptoms of what we called 'manic depression'. It might just be a label, but Dad could expect to go through periods of depression, when he would feel hopeless – as in the wake of his autumn breakdown in 1963. Some of the time, he would seem quite normal. And he would go through other periods when he would feel intensely energetic. This needed to be carefully monitored, as it could get out of hand.

When Dad came back from hospital, there was an uneasy truce for a few months – the phoney war. The university was watching him nervously. His immediate supervisor at the Department of Estate Management since 1962 was a gentle man by the name of John Mills, who quietly suggested that Dad might like to carry on seeing a doctor. The university would, he said, defray the costs. Dad was confused, struggling to come out of his depression. He initially thanked Mills for his concern.

Then Dad's life started to unravel again. On 13 October 1964, he sent out his proposal for the Central Area Shopping

Extension in Cambridge, intended to rejuvenate the neighbourhood. The university authorities had an alternative plan involving a tall tower that Dad deemed a monstrous carbuncle on the face of his beloved city. The day they intended to release their proposal in the media, Dad arranged for four undergraduates with large and garishly coloured helium balloons to float them to where the corners of their proposed building would rise, illustrating the impact on the skyline. So far so good. Looking back on it many years later, I thought it an imaginative and amusing stunt, even if he was rubbing a number of people up the wrong way.

The university did not appreciate the humour. The next day, John Mills put Dad on medical leave. This began the second war of Dad's life, well documented by the missives that flew back and forth, in which Mills played a major role. I immediately wanted to meet him when I read his perceptive and sympathetic letters. Sadly, he was dead, so I had to rely on the written record.

Dad complained to Reverend J. S. Boys Smith, the vice chancellor of the university. 'John Mills's actions are completely contrary to the generally accepted concept of British justice, whereby a person is assumed innocent until proven guilty,' he wrote. Already Dad was using the language of the courts. The allegation of 'illness' was, in Dad's mind, the prosecution's case.

That struck me as ironic. Normally a mental disorder is the case for the defence, the mitigation for whatever might have happened. Dad was taking a better-bad-than-mad approach. Initially, as I read, I had some sympathy with him, because it was not clear what had prompted Mills to act as he had. Mills then made the fifteen-mile drive from Cambridge over to Cheveley Park Stud to seek Mum's cooperation in getting help for her husband. 'Obviously we are sensitive to his breakdown in the summer and autumn of last year when he committed the university to great expense without authority,' he began. 'And he refused my suggestion that he should fully satisfy the university with a medical certificate then.' Now, he explained, Dad appeared to have been picking a very public battle against the people who paid his wages. Dad had been acting strangely, not listening to reason.

'I feel I have to send Dick on leave until I receive from a consultant of the university's choice a certificate that he is fit to carry out duties and responsibilities of the university,' he said carefully. 'It seems to me that the stresses, strains and frustrations that caused that breakdown could well be occurring again following the minister's recent decision on Cambridge planning that differs from Dick's own views.'

My mother was then thirty-eight years old, with three children but little experience of any abnormality of the mind. When Dad had been depressed the year before, she had put it down to exhaustion after a stint of very hard work. We were used to the term 'breakdown' on the stud, since a horse would often break down and not be able to race. A visit from Peter Rossdale, the vet, along with a little rest, and the thoroughbred would be back on the winning track. It was not surprising that Dad was a bit tired again. He was now gadding around doing *three* jobs – he'd taken on the design of a golf course in Ireland, on top of the estate planning and running the stud. Mum knew he might be tired, but it was nothing that a holiday would not cure. She was admirably loyal.

'If you want to make Dick go to a consultant of the university's choice, John, it would seem only fair that at the same time you should visit a consultant of my choosing!' she proposed, with a stridency that was quite unlike her.

'To one knowing nothing of the background, Jean, that might appear fair,' Mills replied. 'I think, however, that in view of last year's events I am right to seek independent advice. I do hope you can help him to see reason, as I very much want him back and doing his very best work.'

He left her to talk it over with her husband. Dad, upon his return, was incensed, the more so when he received the vice chancellor's letter the next day reiterating Mills's demand. The letter was still very cordial, addressed to 'My dear Stafford Smith'. Dad immediately drove over to confront Boys Smith.

'I have discussed the matter fully with my own doctor,' Dad told the vice chancellor. Indeed, Dad had been over to Woodditton House to have a dry sherry with Andrew Dossetor. There was rarely a social event in the Newmarket area where we would not encounter Dr Dossetor and his wife Jill, close family friends. 'You see, he confirms my own view that if, I mean . . . there had been the slightest chink in my mental make-up, it would have been exposed as a result of the pressures to which I have been subjected during the last fortnight or so.'

I began to notice the 'pause phrases' that peppered Dad's language, like 'I mean' and 'you see'. I remember the way he would use those words, making it rather clear that he thought you did not see at all.

'I am afraid, you see,' Dad continued, 'that the production of a medical certificate will only transfer the doubt which exists from me to the person giving the medical advice.'

Boys Smith muttered that this was all very well, but the Financial Board – the curious name they gave to the committee running the university – would be unlikely to settle for anything else. Surely we could agree that a true expert in the profession would be the best way to go? Naturally, the university would expect to pay the bill, and end this disagreeable dispute to the satisfaction of all.

'No, no, Vice Chancellor, this cannot be the way!' Dad replied, his steam rising. 'I mean, professional men, like Christians, can only act on their own judgement and not on other people's. You see, I fear that if you continue to insist on a certificate I will be forced to resign.'

In this line of logic, a 'professional man' like Dad could only be unwell if he felt he was – yet surely even a professional planner would depend on a professional doctor if it were a matter of physical illness. Not so Dad, who walked at top speed from the vice chancellor's office to take the fight to John Mills, where he got no further.

'Look, John, I returned to Cambridge with the firm intention of ensuring as fast as I could within my own professional limitations that the financial position of the colleges was stabilised, you see, and I do not intend giving up this struggle without a fight!' Dad was sounding fairly grandiose here. 'I mean, I believe that the basic character of Cambridge as a university rests with its independent colleges, you see, and I also believe that we are the best people to advise them on property matters.'

'Dick, you keep saying this kind of thing, over and over again,' Mills replied. 'Yet the landslide of letters you have been writing to all and sundry in the university is part of their concern.'

'Frankly, I mean, I believe at the present stage of this tiresome matter "a letter a day keeps the psychiatrists at bay"!'

'I am sorry, Dick,' Mills concluded, after the conversation bounced back and forth across his desk, 'but I must state clearly that I think you are ill and you must remain on leave until such time as you can provide a consultant's certificate that you are fit to resume your duties.'

When he got back to the stud, Dad's sister Jean entered stage left. He had sent her carbon copies of some of his letters, in a sibling spate of self-righteousness.

'Dick, although I am quite aware that you will take no notice of me, you are the son of our mother,' she told him. 'You are both incredibly rude to people.' She gave Dad an elder-sister lecture on how he would achieve much more with honey than vinegar.

Looking back after fifty years, I wondered why he would not just see a shrink and be done with it? When some well-intentioned people raised questions about my own state of mind many years later, I had no qualms about going – though my parsimony rebelled at the cost, and I was disappointed by the unhelpful superficiality of the evaluation. It was at least a useful wake-up call, however. And if Dad genuinely felt there was nothing wrong, he had nothing to fear.

Dr Dossetor was an unfortunate part of the problem. He was my ideal of a family doctor. He came to my bedside every now and then with his black medical bag, sweeping in under the eaves in a waft of carbolic acid, with his braying laugh. He was a steady planet in our family solar system. Yet he was compromised. He'd had some extraordinary experiences – including catching typhus when treating the newly liberated prisoners at the Bergen-Belsen concentration camp – but I don't think he had any particular knowledge of what we call 'mental illness'. It would anyway have been very difficult for him, between eighteen holes of golf with my parents and a quiet game of bridge in the evening, to deliver the long brown envelope of home truths that Dad desperately needed.

Indeed, Dad went over to see him for another glass of sherry.

'The answer to Boys Smith's demand that I see a psychiatrist is that until I know on what grounds the charges against me are based, you see, I am definitely not prepared to undergo a medical examination,' Dad said. 'I mean, it appears now that the university is acting on the advice of its own doctors, who have never seen me and must therefore in turn presumably be acting on second-hand gossip.' Dad was employing more language of the courtroom – not only were they prosecuting him, but they were using hearsay rather than direct evidence. Since he refused to meet with their doctors, however, the university could hardly be faulted.

Andrew Dossetor wondered out loud whether it would not do to just go along with the demand, since he could see nothing wrong with Dad. What did he have to lose?

'If their factual evidence is forthcoming, I mean, maybe we

can consider whether we should give the university a face-saving solution by my going to see someone. But, you see, it will need the very strongest case on their part to persuade me that it is the right step to take.' He drained his glass and shook the doctor's hand as he left. 'In the meantime, Andrew, let me assure you that I shall continue to work a full day as usual!'

This he did – though only in the sense that he was beginning to define 'work' as engaging in endless battles with people who might well have been his allies. Now he went on the offensive in Cambridge, trying to marionette the media. The editor of the local paper had penned an opinion piece referring to Dad as part of the 'Speed Up Group', suggesting that the university was applying conservative brakes. The editorial advocated a 'fusion rather than a confusion of planners', supposing that the people of Cambridge would like them 'knocked together' rather than bickering in public. Dad immediately responded with a long letter about the 'University Plan' and the 'City Plan', prompting a new article the following day clarifying that the City Plan was actually Dad's plan, and had not been supported by the council.

The battle lines were drawn. The deputy treasurer of Cambridge, Dr R. E. MacPherson, wrote to Dad that the Financial Board had formally resolved that he needed to see a psychiatrist of the university's choosing, reminding him that under their rules they might have to consider terminating his employment if he did not provide such a clean bill of health.

'I see that your letter now refers to my "health",' Dad replied, leaping on a semantic point. 'Do I take it that the charge is now being reduced from one of possible madness requiring a psychiatrist's certificate to one of possible physical sickness requiring a certificate of a GP? It is true, incidentally, that I had a slight strain in a shoulder muscle playing tennis two days ago that might explain such a line of attack.'

Physical health, of course, could be the object of humour;

'mental health' could not. Dad resorted to the media with an article about how the university would not meet him and '[his] group'. (To set it in the context of the time, the other front-page reports in the Cambridge paper described Mick Jagger being fined £10 in Wolverhampton for driving without insurance, and a German scientist breaking his silence about how he'd helped to prove that Hitler was dead.) This prompted a further intervention.

Dad had a friend from the social whirl of his Cambridge days, Dr Alice Roughton. She was a psychiatrist known for trying to inject more humanity into the profession – she used to bring her patients home with her to put them back together.

'I was very worried when I saw the *Cambridge News* of Thursday and Friday last week, particularly your letter in Friday's issue,' Alice wrote to him. 'I do not for a moment expect you to agree with me, but I am sure you are not well. As your friend I felt I must let you know what I felt. There are good psychiatrists about, even if you don't believe in them as a race. I know you will tell me the doctors say you are all right – you did before, last year – but I know you, Dick, and you are not all right.'

Dad did not reply, but this was a terrible betrayal. Somehow the enemy had co-opted an old friend to make this stealthy assault upon him from the rear. Even looking back on it, I could not quite see what Dr Roughton had divined from a few letters to the papers. Dad was not playing by the rules of the time – he was not kowtowing to authority – but it was hardly evidence that he needed to be sectioned. If psychosis is very loosely defined as losing touch with reality, that 'reality' is inevitably defined by the norms of a particular society. I delight in prompting people to identify the deranged notions that are accepted without question by 95 per cent of our society today and that will one day be viewed as bizarre. Certainly, many English 'rules' of the early 1960s would be placed far beyond the pale today – from the openly rampant racism to the criminalisation of homosexuality. Perhaps Dad was guilty of no more than biting the hand that was feeding him. Today, we might say he exhibited Asperger's, showing 'significant difficulties in social interaction . . . along with restricted and repetitive patterns of behaviour and interests'. Or we could just say he was being rude. I can imagine Dad feeling intensely alienated, and probably even less inclined to conform.

Either way, the battle of the doctors was creating more problems. Indeed, Dad decided he did need to see another doctor – not to check on his health, but to garner evidence for the defence. Therefore it would be another GP in Newmarket, Dr Anthony Arden-Jones, who wrote the letter that Dad would carry around metaphorically for the next forty years:

Mr Stafford Smith is a rather highly strung, blunt, outspoken individual with a very active mind and a passionate interest in his work. I imagine that he is extremely successful for he has a very fertile brain and is quick to see the important issues in a problem and is obviously fearless and courageous in carrying out any action which he feels to be appropriate in dealing with a problem. I spent a long time examining him, cross-questioning him, and letting him talk. I could find nothing physically wrong with him and thought his mental state was in normal limits. There was absolutely nothing to suggest any serious mental disorder and although at times a little excitable and outspoken, I thought his reaction was completely within the bounds of normality considering the stress to which he has been subjected.

He has reacted to the situation with creditable restraint and forbearance. From what I have heard, Dr Hawtrey-May has never seen Mr Stafford Smith and, as Medical Advisor to the university, this would seem to have been a great mistake.

Hmmm, I thought to myself. It was true that Dr Hawtrey-May had not seen Dad, but that was because Dad still refused to see him. Equally, I doubted Dr Arden-Jones's methodology: the evidence of Dad's 'restraint and forbearance' came from Dad. Arden-Jones did not even talk to my mother, let alone the bevy of concerned citizens queuing up in Cambridge. I wondered how long the doctor had actually spent with Dad. In my own death penalty work, I have had plenty of experience with mental health experts and their fly-by evaluations. Even the better psychiatrists tend to spend no more than two or three hours with one of my clients, which I have always thought far too little – though when I receive their bill at $250 an hour, I sometimes feel it was too long. I felt sure that my father could snow anyone for much longer than that. He believed there was nothing wrong with him and he could, in the words of his sister, prove that black was white and white was black in any argument.

None of the doctors' opinions proved very much as far as I could see. However, there was a pattern that we were going to see escalating for many years thereafter. Dad would be viewed by an increasing number as having a 'mental illness'. He would be confused by this, as he would never see himself as mad. All this achieved in the end was to drive him further and further from those he called colleagues, first, and later from his friends and family.

The university had learned one thing that would take us, as a family, many years to figure out: Dad thrived on his 'letter a day' – and sometimes ten. No matter what you might write, he would reinterpet it, turning around a riposte within hours. But if you just didn't respond, he was reduced to one complaint: you were an ill-mannered lout. In the war of attrition, the university's strategy rapidly devolved into doing nothing. Dad, on the other hand, wanted his job back. Shorn of a responsive enemy, he began to take tentative steps towards seeing some doctor who would satisfy them. He eventually decided he would go down to London to see a respected expert, Dr D. A. Pond.

Dr Pond had done some interesting work in forensics. As early as 1952, he had studied those who killed as part of a pattern of violence, contrasted with those who committed one uncharacteristic violent act. He suggested that the former must have some innate mental flaw which was hardly their fault (this would come under the broad rubric of 'nature'), while the latter seemed to have a dramatic provocation of some kind ('nurture'). Even in those 'hanging' days, the motiveless murderer was treated relatively leniently. 'Of eighteen such cases only two were executed. In five cases the prosecution reduced the charges during the trial to manslaughter. In four cases the prisoners were reprieved after being condemned to death . . . Society is very unwilling to hang such persons,' Pond concluded in an article for the *Journal of Mental Science*. Similarly, with the cases of persistent violence, he said, there is usually no difficulty in finding the defendant diminished in responsibility and suffering from a psychopathic disorder. In other words – heads I win, tails I win: his view was that psychiatry could provide an explanation, and mitigation, for everyone.

Naturally I approved of this, even if his database was rather small. But Dad was concerned with more immediate issues. He lectured Dr Pond in a written preamble to their meeting: 'I do not consider that psychiatric arbitration is the correct medium for resolving this dispute, you see, since I could be perfectly normal mentally and quite incapable of doing my job properly, or mentally abnormal and yet quite capable of performing my duties. I mean, Cambridge is full of examples of both. I am anxious not to give the university or its medical advisors the impression that my attitude has changed on how this extremely tiresome and distressing affair should be decided, because it has not!'

Dr Pond spent a couple of hours with him, and on 10 May

1965 he issued his report. He cut the cake in two, and managed diplomatically to keep everyone relatively happy:

I saw Mr Stafford Smith at the request of his general practitioner. I had a long report from Dr Dossetor, and copies of the letters written by Dr Richard Hunter to the general practitioner when he was treating the patient. There is no doubt that Mr Stafford Smith had an episode in the autumn of 1963 when he was abnormally overactive and excited. This was followed by a period of abnormal depression. Mr Stafford Smith recovered completely from these episodes, but there appears to have been a mild recurrence of symptoms of over-activity and excitement in the autumn of 1964.

When I examined Mr Stafford Smith he seemed to me to be quite normal in mood and I thought that he was fit to return to work. However, in the light of these previous episodes it must be recognised that Mr Stafford Smith is of the manic depressive temperament and there is the possibility that there may be other episodes of either over-excitement or depression. In my view this possibility does not in any way diminish Mr Stafford Smith's capacity to do his job. Now that Mr Stafford Smith himself and all those connected with him in his family and his work are aware that these mood changes can reoccur, it should be possible to take the appropriate measures to get him under treatment at the earliest stages.

As I told Mr Stafford Smith himself, many famous men have suffered from this cyclic temperament. The condition is not progressive, nor associated with any general deterioration.

Dad was happy with this, though ultimately his condition would deteriorate, as he became ever more estranged from all those around him.

The immediate problem had been solved. For the rest of his life, Dad never referred to Dr Pond's diagnosis, and he would deem Dr Hunter's view that he was manic-depressive as 'superseded' by Dr Arden-Jones's assertion that he was completely normal.

That was, in many ways, his tragedy. But it was hardly his fault.

5

Trix, and Growing Up Early

Her wants were few, demands she made of none;
content to smile and welcome in each day.
And yet her life brushed by on many a one
who went the happier on their daily way . . .

Dad's epitaph for his mother, 1972

Back on the Cheveley Park Stud front, Mum was having an increasingly difficult time. Dad had been travelling back and forth to Ireland on the Parknasilla golf project during his enforced holiday from the Department of Estate Management. Even when he was around, he had her type up the reams of spitting letters that the postman took to Cambridge each day. While she had been firmly loyal to him, she was now beginning to see this battle as unwise. At the same time, in the run-up to Christmas 1964, my older brother had been having a psychosomatic inability to sleep. He would be eight on 6 January 1965, and five days later he was slated to go away to boarding school at Old Buckenham Hall (OBH).

Mum had qualms about this. She 'knew' – it was the accepted wisdom – that this was best for Mark, as a private preparatory school was a great privilege that could set him on course to succeed in life. But it had all come very suddenly. It seemed only yesterday that she had finally got her family, and now they were being taken away from her. She worried about Mark. This was not just a couple of nervous nights before going away – he had been an insomniac for weeks, and he was still only seven.

Meanwhile, if she turned round, she was liable to discover that she was being attacked from behind by Granny Smith – Trix. Granny lived in Cheveley Lodge, the big new-brick house protected by another tall brick wall from the children she viewed as 'unscrubbed' in the council houses of the Mansion site. 'Granny gave me this feeling of evilness,' said my sister Mary, years later. Those were strong words for her. I would not use the word 'evil', but when I was young I did not pause to analyse Granny, I just tried to avoid her. Unfortunately, she often used to summon me over to churn her milk, a chore that gave me a lifetime loyalty to Anchor butter, imported from far-away New Zealand.

Every Sunday, Trix would come over for lunch. She would berate us for our bad manners, and moan about the slightest spot on 'her' dining room chairs – ugly red leather monstrosities she had given my parents. She was devoted to expensive things. If she was going to be seen in town, or at the races, she wrapped herself in her fox bolero, on top of her mink coat.

Mark, the firstborn son, was favoured. She mostly tolerated me. Mary, though, she would constantly put down, saying how much better the boys were at things. Still, her primary hostility was reserved for Mum, who was just not good enough for her only son.

'I eventually worked out that Granny had some strange desire to keep up the emotional pinpricks until I cried,' Mum explained. 'As soon as I cried she would stop, so I learned to cry as soon as possible as that would bring it to an end.' She could not avoid the sharp points altogether.

In retrospect, I now see that Granny was miserable in her Midasian cage. She had been alone in her marriage to her gay husband, and cut off from her true background since, although I have inherited her rather stereotypical Jewish nose myself, she would never have countenanced the fact. She was overtly hostile to her sister Ve's husband, the raucous Uncle Fenny, who was a diminutive and (to her anti-Semitic eye) embarrassingly Jewish bookmaker. Now widowed, two miles up the avenue that led to the stud, she was lonely.

It was July 1966, the World Cup final. I remember people crammed into the sitting room watching the black-and-white television at my maternal grandparents' home in Fordham. For many, it was a rerun of the Second World War, just twenty-one years on from VE Day. It was the first and last time I saw my mother show any interest in football.

Dad was evolving, and the signs were troubling. Even though the letter from Dr Pond had met the university's demands, he had resigned. Despite having a stud to run, and the golf course project in Ireland, he took on consultancy work for Leslie 'Bill' Bilsby, who ran a construction company called SPAN. Bill loved a good argument as much as Dad, and his nineteen-year-old daughter, my godmother Caroline, was a witness to one of their debates. Her parents had brought her up in a conservative Methodist tradition where the Trinity of the Father, the Son and the Holy Ghost were clearly defined, and she was rather taken aback when Dad announced that he was Jesus Christ reincarnated.

Bill was a sincere Christian, and she expected her father to raise an objection. He did not. Perhaps Dad was making a debating point in his typically outlandish way, but Caroline was left confused: Dad could be charismatic – perhaps it was time for the Second Coming, and who was to say that it could not take place in East Anglia, around the time England also won the World Cup?

It might have been better if Bill had simply laughed at Dad, whose mania was on the rise. Bill's business dealings with the Suffolk Saviour did not last very long: Dad had presented a plan for a Science Town not far from Cambridge to the local residents, and when this crashed in the face of intense opposition, rather than backing off he planned ten more. It was one thing for Dad to take over running the world as the Son of God, but SPAN had to make a profit.

Early the following summer, I had an experience I remember vividly. It was evening, but still daylight. Dad told me to come with him into the lounge. 'Now, Clive,' he began, 'I want to talk to you about where you are in life.' The primary issue in my mind was my eighth birthday coming up on 9 July; I hoped for various presents. Dad was not interested in that. He explained that when he was very young he had been required to fight for his country. He had, he said, persuaded his mother – Granny Smith – to help him sign up before he was really old enough, and he had gone off to war. I knew the story. He said he had been sixteen, which was a pretty advanced stage in evolution as far as I was concerned.

'The big problem you face these days, Clive, is that society is trying to keep you immature,' he opined. 'You understand what that means? It means that you just aren't prepared for the world, you see. And, I mean, that is not good for you. So I had this idea. Here, I am giving you two hundred pounds.' He handed me a pile of banknotes, an unimaginable amount. At the time, our pocket money was twice our age in pennies each week – this was before decimalisation, so that meant I got fourteen pence, or a shilling and tuppence. I was looking forward to it going up to one and fourpence in just a few days. Dad had just handed me about sixty-six years of pocket money. That was pretty exciting, but I was worried that there was a catch.

'So this is the agreement,' Dad continued. 'I give you this money – lend it really, as you'll have to pay it back in the end, you see. But there's no interest to be paid on it. And you have a choice. I mean, you can either stay here if you pay rent, and we'll agree how much you have to pay. Or you can choose to go live where you like, and pay your own way. This money ought to last you a while, but you'll have to start planning on how to make the money you need when it comes to an end.'

I was confused. I wasn't sure what 'lending' was. I had no

idea what he meant by 'interest'. I had only the vaguest idea of what 'rent' might be. I was slightly concerned about paying to stay in my bedroom, as I imagined that there were a lot of collateral considerations, perhaps involving the status of my teddy bears.

Naturally, Dad had not talked to Mum about this idea. She came into the lounge as Dad was finishing and she figured out what was happening. She gently took me into the hall, prised the money from my hand, told me not to worry and sent me up to bed. What she said to Dad thereafter I can only guess.

Ironically, just a few weeks later, they would kick me out of the house anyway, as they had Mark, but they would give the money to someone else.

If you raise the issue of boarding school with a man who went to one at the age of seven or eight, he will give you one of two reactions. Either 'It was the making of me, and look how successful I am today!' Or, after some prevarication, you might elicit an admission that he is currently a member of the 'Survivors of Boarding School'.

It is a shame that both camps are so defensive, and sometimes so overtly traumatised. I did not really think about school until nearly fifty years later; it was just a part of my past. Between the ages of eight and thirteen, I lived most of my life at Old Buckenham Hall. Had you asked me a few years ago about life at OBH, I would have said, yes, it had been a little difficult at first, and I had been homesick, but ultimately I had been the most privileged of the privileged. I became head boy (as my brother had been before me), I played all the sports, I had a couple of truly influential teachers, the headmaster invited me back for an extra week of Latin to ensure that I could get a scholarship to Radley College, and so forth – I was very fortunate.

Had I got carried away in the pompous manner I learned at boarding school, I might indeed have said that it was the 'making of me'. I had no insight into its emotional impact on me – indeed, I lacked it for decades. This reminds me not to be too harsh in my criticism when Dad, and those around him, failed to see his own idiosyncrasies.

When I went to the unfamiliar environment of OBH, I missed my family, my home, my teddies, and the little mouse who used to scurry around my bedroom. I blubbed – that dreadful prep-school word – every night for the first month. Some years later, my mother tried her hand at writing a book of letters to an imaginary friend. Each missive began 'Dear Betty', and described life on a Newmarket stud. Mum's imagined mother had only two children, one called Philippa (clearly my sister Mary) and the other Adrian (me). Adrian is my middle name, and Dad had wanted to call me that but fortunately Mum vetoed it on the grounds that I would have gone through life with 'ASS' for my initials. 'Adrian is very happy at his prep school, though he was "unusually" (to quote the headmaster) homesick when he first went,' she wrote to Betty. 'His first letter was pathetic – "the only good thing about this school is sleep" . . .'

I must have managed to get a degree of my heartache into my letters home, which was surprising. We wrote home each week at a set time on Friday evening, in a series of 1950s brick classrooms, with iron-framed windows, that ran down a colonnade from the main OBH mansion house to the pine-floored gymnasium where we had assembly every day. The entire school would be required to reassure parents that their money was being well spent. When we had completed a letter, we had to hand it in – it was reviewed for length and for content.

In other words, it was censored – much like the correspondence from the men I would later represent in Guantánamo Bay. If we inserted anguish, the consequences would be explained to us. *It will only upset your mother if you say that, and she is not here, so she will worry.* You would be given a new sheet of paper. This was a lesson about emotion; it was vital that you should *lie*. If you told the truth, it brought trouble in two ways: you would be chastised for causing suffering, and you would have to start over rather than go out to play football. Sometimes the teacher was slovenly (bored of reviewing 'I hope you are well, I am' scratched in pencil by 120 students) and misery would seep through.

Mum must have brought it up with Donald Sewell, the headmaster, given the reference to me being 'unusually' homesick. That was a cover-up on his part, as the sobbing in the dormitory was contagious. By the third letter, the censor had been instructed to be more attentive. 'His next letter,' Mum wrote to Betty, 'thank goodness, went, "I am almost settled in now. I am *quite* happy now."'

For the first couple of terms, I slept in a small dormitory at the top of the eyrie tower far above the junior dining room. Some boys strove to show fortitude – Mark, for example. I remember him for his derring-do, standing on the bed next to the window grinning demonically as he threw his own shit out. But most of us would sneak under the cold sheet and the rough brown blanket and 'blub' when the lights went out.

There were several moments of particular misery in the diary: foremost, the return to school after holidays or half-term. Next, the curiously defined 'long weekend' and two 'short' weekends. Each Sunday, rain or shine, we would walk a mile to Thorpe Morieux church and endure an hour-long service with a tedious sermon. On a short weekend, parents could pick up their children after the service, around eleven o'clock, and pupils would spend five hours out on parole. It was not worth driving home, so we would end up going for lunch in Lavenham, and then perhaps move directly on to tea somewhere else, before returning to school. The long weekends were worse: we were allowed to skip church, so we had a full seven hours. After the twenty-six miles home (which took an hour back then) and Sunday lunch, there was time to notice everything about home that seemed so achingly familiar before driving back.

I never conquered homesickness, though I sequestered it into a small corner of my chest. Thinking about it now, I can feel the creeping chill of dread as we headed up the drive towards the school. The kids who were not able to force it to one side were the overtly wretched ones, yet even this was not the most insidious impact of being 'sent away'.

In 1967, my nascent idea of love had been home, where Vesta the black Labrador wagged her tail in welcome each morning, I could always look to my older sister for advice (Mark would be in the bedroom with a science-fiction book), and it only took a phone call to get my best friend Anthony over to play all day. I was fine going to primary school, with Mum driving us the five minutes into Newmarket and picking us up at three each afternoon.

The notion of being sent away at eight seemed hateful. Yet Mum explained to me that they were paying a substantial sum to make it possible, because they loved me. This, then, was what 'love' really meant. Either they were right or I was. For a child there can be only one answer: love was not the cocoon of home, it was 'maturing' far away. Rather than get a reputation as a blubber, I had to toughen up.

Once I had internalised the basic lesson that love meant separation, a number of logical consequences flowed. Engulfing love was to be avoided, because it would end in tears when the other person thrust me away. I should strive to be a self-sufficient island. The best way to achieve that was to learn to dissociate from my feelings. When some troubling emotion bubbled up, I should inspect it, remember my lesson and lock it away. I should do the same to any emotion – love, fear, hate or anger.

Prep school also came with the standard physical abuses. I got beaten more than most, almost exclusively for talking after lights out. This inclined me to deride authority: if masters employed their harshest punishment on me for telling a story to my friends, the challenge was to find a way around them. I would never snitch on another boy and I expected them to live by the Code as well – we were conditioned to sneak around authority, and to lie if we were caught. I do wonder whether our superfluity of boarding-schooled members of parliament have had the therapy necessary to recognise this in themselves; after all, it took me long enough.

The idea of thrashing a child for discipline is an extraordinary one, and it has happily been outlawed. At the time, I once complained to Dad that the school shouldn't do it.

'I send you away to school,' he said, 'because I don't have the courage to beat you myself.' Looking back, he probably meant he would never beat me, but that was not the way I took it. Love was, I thought, about making sure someone was beaten.

By the age of twelve I didn't do emotion any more. This must have been a benefit back when the boarding school boy was sent alone to India to 'run the Raj'. In the 1970s it was less useful. I did not understand it then, but somehow I had to take my own idiosyncrasies and work out a way in which they could help in life, rather than hinder. With pure fortuity, I suppose I was successful at doing that, at least insofar as my profession was concerned. I have had to witness six clients – human beings for whom I cared – being tortured to death a few feet in front of me after I failed to stop their executions. Perhaps that would be an intolerable experience for some, but I was able to dissociate and let the portcullis rattle down. I could still see what was happening through the criss-crossed iron bars, but I was securely protected.

At prep school I was taught to sneer internally at the 'wet' boys; later, I was guilty of thinking less of lawyers who 'burned out' in the cauldron of capital litigation. Did they not understand? They were weak. They were not the victims of the gas chamber, the electric chair or the gurney. That 'privilege' was reserved for our clients.

However, I was also, I suspect, a stranger to that emotion some people call 'love' – throughout life, at least until my son was born. I suspect I did not understand love at all, no matter all the poems I wrote. This was a deficit I shared with Dad. He would write lengthy tracts for us about the definition of love, but it was all an intellectual discussion. Like me, Dad had had the emotion and empathy squashed out of him, but I don't remember him having any insight into this deficit – any more than the boarding school boys in the British cabinet seem to today.

6

The Game of Happy Families Is Over

And on the pedestal, these words appear:
'My name is Ozymandias, king of kings,
Look on my works, ye Mighty, and despair.'
Percy Bysshe Shelley, 'Ozymandias'

As I neared the end of my time at prep school, my dad would regale me with stories about how well the stud was going; he increasingly believed that he had a formidable ability to judge the value of a horse. Forlorn River, who Dad had bought for £25,000, was the proof of his Midas touch. I accepted his press release on our best stallion, who came to us after winning the 1967 July Cup and the Nunthorpe Stakes.

Forlorn River 'stood' at the stud, in equine language, and mares would 'visit'. The 'covering' took place in a barn in the stallion yard, from which the stallion man would, in a rather prudish way, try to banish my sister Mary, although as the future biologist she was much more interested than I was. It was vital to time the covering carefully. The gestation period of a horse is usually 330 to 345 days, depending on the mare. The earlier a foal is born in the year, the more mature the horse will be when it comes time for the thoroughbred's sole purpose, which is racing; but strive too hard, and disaster strikes. All thoroughbreds in the northern hemisphere have a 'birthday' on New Year's Day (in the southern hemisphere it is 1 August), so if a foal is born on 31 December, the animal will be one year old the next day. Horses start competing at two, and since many races are designated for two-year-olds only, such an animal will really be a yearling when competing, the equivalent of a child running against students twice her age.

Every mare has a 'foal heat' when she has a foal at foot, seven to twelve days after giving birth. If you want to get a foal out of a mare each year – and your investment may demand this – that is when she needs to be in the covering yard. This is a notion that must send shudders down the spine of any woman who has just come through childbirth.

Once or twice a year, I ventured over to watch the marvel of a foal being born. Peter Rossdale, the vet, would be there amid the straw, with a red heat lamp warming the winter stable. He would pull on an extraordinary plastic glove that extended almost to his shoulder, and then, standing directly in line with her kicking hooves, reach deep into the mare to help her give birth. The foal would appear, head tucked between the two front legs, enclosed in the bluish-white amniotic sac. The mare would lick her offspring and, within minutes, the little beast would be teetering up on spindly legs, in extraordinary contrast to the first experiences of human newborns.

Nationally, Forlorn River was the leading sire for his first crop – meaning that he had come to Cheveley Park in 1967, sired some forty foals in 1968, and these did particularly well racing as two-year-olds in 1970. Mary used to pore over the form book, and had modest results from a £1 bet every now and then. I was very suspicious of gambling, which I saw as a trail of torn-up betting slips. (The perils of the industry are starkly illustrated by the fact that, in 2006, a promising American two-year-old called the Green Monkey was auctioned for a record $16 million. Two years later, after no victories in three starts and with career winnings of only $10,440, he was officially retired to begin what turned out to be an unsuccessful stud career.)

I don't think any of us understood it at the time, but Dad could not have picked a less appropriate profession than the 'racing industry', given his temperament. With his mounting mania, gambling was not a good bet. If you stand near the track, a racehorse thundering past the rail may seem very vital, but the reality of horse breeding is that nothing else moves fast. Even in flat racing, there are many fences between the stallion sperm bank and the finish line – the complex interrelation between sire and dam, the time of year the horse is born, the trainer, the jockey, when it last rained, the drainage of the soil, and even the horse's will to win. Mary was a patient biologist, and she loved horses. Dad may have admired the animals, but that was his only obvious qualification.

Two years after Forlorn River had his first successful crop, Dad told Mary of an offer that had just been made on the horse – £400,000, or sixteen times what he had paid.

'What do you think?' he asked. 'Should we accept it?'

Mary thought about it seriously – I can see her creased brow, as she considered most things very seriously – though not for very long. 'I think you should definitely take it,' she said with emphasis. Dad had started borrowing large sums from Barclays Bank to 'improve' the stud; she explained how he could pay off the debt and have plenty left over to buy two or three more stallions with the skill he said he had developed.

Dad's face darkened. So many of Dad's 'discussions' were actually a search for validation: there was no way he was going to part with his precious horse, and he was angry at Mary for disagreeing with a decision he had already made. To him, Forlorn River was worth far more.

Auntie Jean was cynical about it. 'I gather Forlorn River is worth a million now,' she said. 'What sweet dreams are made of!' Dad rounded on her as well: she was just a woman, with a 'middle-class mind'. Indeed, he was picking fights with anyone in his vicinity. He wrote a letter to the *Sporting Life* describing how the average stud hand was making seventeen pounds, five shillings a week, plus a tied cottage worth perhaps four pounds, and a fuel allowance of thirty shillings. Annually this amounted to a little over £1,000 or so. Though he did not put it in so many words, they were paid less than the value of one vial of Forlorn River's semen. At £35 a week, owners paid more to board a mare at the stud than we paid the staff.

Lieutenant Colonel Douglas Gray was running Hadrian Stud, and he called Dad up, interested in taking the discussion forward. 'In my view,' he opined, 'my men are well paid in comparison to other jobs in the agricultural sphere.'

'You're wrong on that,' Dad replied. 'I mean, first, it's not a normal agricultural job – the men have to look after incredibly valuable animals. And second, it's very hard, and I'd venture to bet that you wouldn't like to do it in all weathers and take home the pay packet which they take home.'

'Are you saying I'm not capable of doing what my men do?' the colonel bridled. 'I will tell you, I have led men into places you have never been . . .'

'I didn't say you couldn't, I said you wouldn't,' Dad said, turning up the volume. 'I mean, you obviously think you're talking to some sort of revolutionary, whilst I feel I'm talking to a cross between an idiot and an old woman.'

'I think you should withdraw what you just said!'

'I'm not going to withdraw anything!' Dad was very loud by now. 'You see, I am a person who says what he means, and means what he says. I think your attitude belongs somewhere in the worst period of the nineteenth century rather than what one might hope to be the more enlightened century we are currently in.'

Dad may well have been correct – the staff were underpaid – but none of the money he was borrowing was going towards increasing their wages. Auntie Jean had previously pointed out that Dad, like his mother, could be just rude, but it was unclear to me what he expected to gain from it. What did his response say about his state of mind? Social norms set certain boundaries. My own profession is contentious, yet I have always been taken aback when some prosecutor becomes overtly aggressive. It is such an odd way to behave if you want to persuade another person.

After I read Chinua Achebe's book *Things Fall Apart*, the title swirled around in my head. I find it descriptive of various stages of life – and certainly the moment when my family's idyll at Cheveley Park Stud began to fragment. It had begun when we were sent away to school. Then Dad lost interest in the daily routine of running the stud, and it became an asset for his larger ambitions. The end for Mum came in 1972, with the so-called Cocks Affair.

Dad liked to barter – rather than paying for a car with filthy lucre, he would 'do work' for Cocks Garage in Cambridge and receive a new Triumph Vitesse in return. Perhaps there was once an era when this worked, but the fly in Dad's economic ointment was that he rated the value of his work far higher than did others. He had not paid for his latest car and the company had repeatedly said he must; he took it in for a service and they, relying on the adage that possession was nine-tenths of the law, refused to return it until he paid his bill.

There had been a conversation back at home, and Mum had tried to explain to us that there was a dispute over fees. Mark suggested that it would be more gentlemanly to pay up and argue over the money later.

'Dad was awful to Mark . . .' Mum told me years later. 'This was not what family loyalty was all about.' He made Mark go with him in one of the stud vehicles to the garage, located where the Newmarket Road runs into Cambridge, and told him he had to climb into the dealership. Mark refused. He said it was stealing, and that he had been brought up not to steal. Dad retorted that it was his filial duty. Mark turned and walked away, in the middle of the night, in a city fifteen miles from home. When his roiling emotions were sufficiently in check, he started looking for a telephone box. 'I had to rescue him,'

Mum said. She left Mary and me in bed, and drove off into the darkness in search of her oldest child in her green Ford estate.

Somehow, Dad managed to extricate the sports car himself. The following morning, we were meant to be driving to Cornwall on a camping holiday, and Mum decided she had a duty to talk to him. Just as I would later give Mary licence to intercede for me in respect of my own welfare if it were ever necessary, when Dad had his breakdown in 1963 he and Mum had agreed that she should tell him when he was off the rails. It must have been an awful prospect for her. It would have been difficult for Dad as well. He was about to be told he was losing touch with his mind. Could there be anything worse?

He was in the bath. When he was manic, he would take as many as four baths a day, as if it would help to wash away his tension. It was a sign we came to recognise.

Mum squatted down, talking to him on the level. 'Look, darling, I owe it to you to suggest that you need a little medical assistance,' she began tentatively. 'I am not suggesting you are "round the bend" as you put it, but I do have a desire not to see you continually blocking your own opportunities for great achievement.'

Dad looked back at her without saying anything. It had been a long night – he hadn't got home until the early hours. It was rare for her to get the chance to speak without interruption – he must have been taken aback. So she went on.

'I have always had such faith in your ability . . . so do the children. You have such brilliant ideas, such potential. Just look at the number of people who are infected with your enthusiasm and ideas . . . and then? What becomes of the wonderful schemes you propose?'

However kindly put, Mum was essentially telling him that all his plans were coming to nothing: he was failing, failing, failing.

'I hope you know I have always been prepared to help unstintingly. But this week has been the worst you've ever been.' She paused. She needed to let him have some excuse – the 'exhaustion' from overwork that had allegedly precipitated his earlier breakdown. 'I am sure you have many problems on your mind, I don't know, but honestly you don't seem to know whether you're coming or going. And most of all, in the current state you are in, you have lost your ability to convince people. You had me type up that letter you wanted to send to Lord Rothschild. It was the rudest letter I can ever remember you writing – and I'll eat some hay or whatever if you've had a favourable response to it.'

By now, Dad's look was as cold as his bath. The bubbles had all burst.

'I suppose I could keep my head in the sand,' Mum said. 'But I cannot sit by with Mark's tears. He's still paralysed by what you told him to do. I know you think he let you down, and in terms of unquestioning faith he did, but you taught him so many things – to question people, and to do what he thinks is honest. You may not notice, but he does little things to help you all the time. He so achingly wants to be your friend.

'There was a time when you had trusted me if I said you needed a holiday . . . But then you began not to listen to me, so I gave up – too easily, perhaps. Maybe I have let you down, but I want you to know that there was a poem you gave me once – "Anchorage" – which I value most above all else you've ever written.'

Dad was a great one for quoting poetry. Mum rarely indulged, but she had the creased paper with her, showing how often she had looked at it. I can only imagine what it took for her to get the words out, while Dad was silently seething.

Where our summer loves desert us, and flatterers turn to foes,
  When memories only hurt us, and dreams augment the blows;

74

When dependency lurks beside us and the night seems pit-like black;

Who have we then to guide us, and point the sure road back?

Some set the course through shifting sand, alone to the bitter end.

Thank God I felt a helping hand, and turning, found a friend!

She paused. He was staring up at the ceiling.

'Darling, won't you please accept my love and that of the whole family?' she finished. She stooped to kiss him on the forehead as she left. He did not move. She found herself trembling with emotion.

The three of us – Mark, Mary and me – were finishing up breakfast in the kitchen. Dad got out of the bath and dressed. He came to the bottom of the stairs in the hall, as we were taking things out to the car, packing up to go.

He said he wanted everyone in the lounge, now. 'You can stop that packing,' he said sternly, whereupon he waited until we were all seated on the gold-upholstered sofa.

'Your mother thinks that I am mad, mentally deranged, you see. Apparently . . . because I told Mark that family duty required him to help me right a wrong . . . So you now have a choice. I mean, you can go to Cornwall with your mother, or you can stay here and support me. This is the moment, I am afraid, that you have to choose me or your mother.' He paused for a long moment. We were all very confused. Mum, I am sure, was trying to work out what to say. He then concluded – and the words reverberate down to me over many decades – 'If you go with her now . . . you needn't expect to see me ever again.'

I don't remember what Mum did at that moment. I have a sense that she was standing helplessly behind the three of us.

Mark got up silently, walked out of the room, passed through the big glass door from the hall to where Mum had backed the car up to be packed, and sat in the passenger seat waiting to go. Mary followed him.

I was bewildered, but it was black or white, one thing or the other. I thought he was telling me that it was the last time I would ever see him. I took him literally.

'Well, if you're telling me I have to choose, I'll go with Mum then, I suppose,' I said eventually, looking first up at him, and then at Mum.

That took the wind rather out of his sails for a moment. Mum ushered me out of the room to the car. We all got in, leaving him standing there as Mum drove away. My impression is that he was forlorn.

Mark cried all the way to Cornwall. 'That was the moment I decided I had to divorce Dad,' Mum said later. Mark was still crying on the second day, after we had stopped overnight at a relative's. 'The clutch was slipping the whole way,' she added.

It was a miserable holiday. We camped on the farm of some extended family, the Boadens, at Porthleven. It seemed to rain the entire two weeks. We had our old orange family tent – and also, for the first time, the luxury of a separate toilet tent with a hole dug into the sodden field. It blew up towards the gloomy clouds while I was in there. The surrounding cows, taken aback as much as I was, stared ruminatively at me.

Then there was the dreadful visit to the Minack outdoor theatre, an astounding venue carved into the cliff – I would normally have marvelled at it. We watched a play, long forgotten but for the moment when an actor held out his hand and intoned, 'I think I feel a spot of rain!' Cold rainwater had been dribbling down the neck of my windcheater throughout the performance.

The fortnight was all the more incomprehensible to me since Dad did show up more than once in Cornwall. He had sworn that I would never see him again, yet here he was already, jovial and pretending to play happy families. He drove from London each time, and though he was a maniacal driver it must have taken him six hours. He would arrive around noon, leaving before evening – to return, as Mum knew though I did not, to his lover and erstwhile secretary, Dawn, in his flat on Park Lane. Mum later told me she would have forgiven him that, but she could not get past what he had done to Mark.

7

Nouveau Riche, Nouveau Pauvre

It is estimated that 70% of wealthy families will lose their
wealth by the second generation and 90% will lose it by the
third.

Nasdaq Personal Finance, 2019

Dad used to say of my mother's family, unkindly, that the first
generation makes it, the second keeps it and the third loses it.
He was right: Great-Uncle Allen was an entrepreneur and set
up a thriving ready-mixed concrete company; my godfather
Jeremy was a man of *noblesse oblige* privilege who would rather
cut off his right hand than sack an employee; my third-
generation cousin seemed to think he had a genetic right to
inherit a supremely well-paid job (for which he was manifestly
ill-suited). He drove the company inexorably towards the
receivers.

I never plucked up the courage to point out to my father
that, on the paternal side, my grandfather had made his fortune
(in the form of Robert Sherwood's bequest) and Dad blew it,
without allowing my siblings and me the chance to do so.

Auntie Jean was exhausted from dealing with Dad at this
point, and she wanted out of the stud. Her first idea, generous
in spirit, caused all kinds of trauma. She suggested that she just
pass on her interest in the stud for roughly what it might have
been worth when her father died, perhaps £40,000. Dad should
pay for it, but it should be in our names: though inevitably, that
was not how Dad chose to interpret her proposal.

I was twelve. Dad wrote to each of us telling us that we had to raise this money, the equivalent of a little over half a million pounds today. 'Auntie Jean has now asked that she be released from acting as co-trustee and be bought out of her reversionary interest in the stud assets,' he began, using a series of words I had to look up in the dictionary. 'She has also asked that it should be purchased by you three, you see, and that after Granny's death (which we all hope will be a long time hence) the stud will belong half to me and one sixth each to each of you. I mean, this is a very nice idea of Auntie Jean's and I hope in due course you will write and tell her so.' I wasn't really interested in owning a stud, though I was happy to be living there.

A few days later, I wrote back to Dad about borrowing my share, or £13,333.

'Dear Dad,' I scratched. My handwriting was more legible than Mark's, but fell far short of the beautiful lines of Mum's script, or even Mary's. 'To tell the absolute truth I do not understand the full implication of it. Although I am out of my depth, I am quite sure I do not trust the theory. If you can persuade me, all right, but it will be a hard job as I am very suspicious of money by nature. See you sometime. Love, Clive.'

I included a scrappy worksheet where I had done my calculations by some complicated use of logarithms, since I had not yet been allowed a calculator. I was assuming 8 per cent fixed annual interest, so servicing my part of the debt would cost me £1,066.64 a year. Dad assured me I would somehow receive £1,000 income, but I figured I would have to pay 30 per cent in taxes, which meant I lost £366.64 a year. This was a staggering amount. Decimalisation had upped my pocket money to 26p a week, yet it would still take me a quarter-century to pay off one year's loss.

I added a sad postscript: 'You don't have to be in the Fathers' cricket match if you do not want to. I probably shall not be in it.' I would have loved to play in the match, as cricket was my passion, but I was giving him an out as I did not think he would come. Three years before, Dad had stripped off his jacket to take part in a fathers' race; I can still hear the sound of the change jangling in his pocket, and feel the pride with which I watched him rushing up the track. I don't remember now whether he won – it was the taking part, the only time he did.

By now, Mum was finding it increasingly difficult to keep three children in private school. She periodically sent Dad demands for help with the school fees, which he normally ignored and never paid. He would make an occasional grand entrance. Once, he arrived at the stud in a helicopter, which he had commandeered to take Mary back to Queenswood, the boarding school Mum was somehow financing. I was home at the time, and I went up for a ride. I had been eyeing the single main rotor, wondering aloud just how safe these things were. The pilot winked at me and simply turned the engine off. We settled down to the ground as if we were a seed from a syca-more tree.

Dad had reduced Mary's housemistress to tears several times, so the poor woman had been replaced on this occasion by Miss Seal, who was tough enough to handle him. Mary, he com-plained in one of his periodic missives to the school, was not getting a proper *feminine* education. 'As I have often told her, the first duty of all human beings in society is to be attractive both physically and emotionally to those with whom they are going to mix. One of the fundamental requirements, then, is to "feminise" Mary, otherwise she undoubtedly will be a lesbian by the time she is twenty-five,' he wrote.

'This may or may not be a bad thing in the long run, but it certainly does not help for either the happiness or fulfilment in the present state of English society. She told me this morning that she is playing in the hockey trials,' he continued, in scan-dalised tones. 'Hockey has, of course, done more harm for the female character in England than any other single factor as not only does it develop the most unfeminine muscles, but it also develops a number of unfeminine characteristics. You will gather that this has confirmed my view that Queenswood is among the most ineffectual, negative and dangerous institutions in the whole educational field. Unfortunately, the level of maturity among most of those teaching at the school is appallingly low. I explained to Mary that the reason I was keen for her to stay on was that I thought she might be able to help the situation.'

He copied me in to all this. At the time, I thought it was how people behaved with each other. Some of my portentous essays that survive from school reflect his influence.

I knew Dad was totally serious. Mary was aiming for A levels in physics, chemistry and biology. It did not matter what she did, in his eyes she was doomed to lose. Either she was dedicated to science and was therefore a lesbian, or she was not taking enough maths and was therefore not as logical as her brothers. She was, in one way, much better equipped to deal with Dad than I was, since she had not been sent away to school until she was eleven, and therefore suffered less emotional scarring from this source at least. But she was also at a disadvantage, since perhaps she did not have the exoskeleton that was designed to keep emotions well under cover.

Dad's mood continued to slope up and down throughout 1972. Auntie Jean was not sure whether to worry more when he was depressed or when he appeared to be cheering up.

'I have managed to decipher Dick's letter, which fills me with the direst gloom,' she wrote to Mum – they were both experts in reading his illegible scrawl. 'He is obviously feeling only too much better, and full of plans. It is a mystery how anyone can think of buying more stud farms when the one they already have is losing money despite it being in a prime situation and well equipped. If he ends up in jail, that is his affair.'

Dad was on the Continent, buying horses, some of which he dispatched back to the stud where they were meant to be fed and stabled. One mare arrived from his latest adventure in Holland, and Peter Rossdale gave her the once-over. She had a heart defect, he said, and might drop dead at any moment. He suggested that it might make sense to do a thorough check-up before handing the money over. Another mare, Native Honey, came seventh out of twenty in a minor race, but Dad wrote that she should stay in training at £1,000 a year – roughly what we paid the stud hands – as she would doubtless win a race or two. She never did.

When the borrowing reached about £180,000, Barclays Bank asked for it to be reduced. Naturally, Dad decided to increase his debt instead. He came up with a Cayman Island diversion to restructure the Barclays money, setting up some fiscal shenanigans with a bank there. He then remortgaged the stud with the Agricultural Mortgage Corporation for an addititional £240,000 at 9 per cent interest. He was now £400,000 in debt – well over £3 million in today's money.

Using some of the new funds, Dad bought Dawn a flat in Rosas, north of Barcelona. Mum had encouraged Mary and me to visit him there while he was recovering from a bout of hepatitis that he had picked up swimming in the Mediterranean. He was quite excitable, I thought, though at this stage I had no understanding of his illness. When Mary and I expressed our concerns about the borrowing, Dad explained his theory.

'It's a mug's game, don't you see?' he said. 'The money is borrowed at 9 per cent. Inflation this year is running at 16 per cent. So if I do no more than keep up with inflation, I make 7 per cent. And what's 7 per cent of £400,000?'

He turned to me, as he had some fixation that I was a maths machine. That one was rather easy: £28,000.

'Right, you see, so we get £28,000 for doing nothing. And, I mean, that is only the beginning. I predict that inflation is going to rise to 25, 30 per cent in the next few years, and I have the borrowing fixed. And I can make much more, maybe a 50 per cent return. You see what I mean? It's a mug's game!'

Initially, my young mind could not see any flaws in his logic. I did not know how fast Dad could drain money away: if he bought a flat for Dawn, for instance, that was not factored into the profit. His expenses soared when he was excitable. He was now negotiating an additional loan of £60,000 from the AMC at 16 per cent. Mum found it all depressing. The stud had been worth a million pounds and yet there was nothing in the account.

'I cannot get neurotic over money,' she said to Auntie Jean, 'so I find it hard to fight tooth and nail for it. But at the same time it is heartbreaking to see your heritage and Dick's being swallowed up in this mess of pottage.' Mum was a curious mixture when it came to finances. On one level, she was extremely careful. In part because of her emphatic indoctrination, I have reached sixty years old without ever paying a single penny in interest to a credit card company. They are simply usurers, she would say, and I learned at an early age what compounding interest meant. Yet at the same time Mum was very generous. Her other mantra was that if you were ever asked for a loan, you should do it if you could, but only on the understanding that it did not have to be repaid – that way, you never got into disputes with friends over what they owed you.

The banks took a rather different view. Dad managed to put up everything Mum owned as collateral for his loans.

'Have you been told you have a middle-class mind?' poor Auntie Jean asked her. 'He must have said that to me fifty times in the last two days. I told him he was only saying that because he has a monumental inferiority complex which makes him put other people down. In the past, he has admitted that is true, but only when he's down. He's not saying that right now.'

Meanwhile, Dad refused Jean's entreaty to stop buying horses. 'He has a new idea where he will transfer the debt to Spain where the interest rate is only 6 per cent,' she continued despondently. 'He insists that Rapid River and Melchbourne are brilliant, and Souvran will be even better.' These were to be the heirs to the sperm-bank money machine, Forlorn River.

Pondering this later in life, I realised why I dislike banks.

They insist that they oil the wheels of capitalism, yet they do not pause to think what is best for the individuals they claim to serve. If morality is indeed a matter of motive, as Dad always insisted, then banks are a moral black hole, their true motive only to make more money.

Dad was high as a kite. Mum and Jean had no means of curbing his spendthrift ways; the banks had total control over Dad's ability to spend money. Dad had no realistic plans, yet the banks ignored the consequences of their actions, so long as their 'investment' was secured by the stud, by life insurance policies, and ultimately by the house to which Mum might be able to retreat with her children.

Like my mother, I have no personal interest in whether my family should have hung on to my grandfather's random inheritance. After all, we had become nouveau riche with the allocation of the stud to my grandfather Albert by Bob Sherwood, so there was no real loss if we became nouveau pauvre – a very relative term, since we were all raised in immense privilege. But that did not excuse the banks, who were facilitating not just Dad's self-destruction but also his increasingly cruel mistreatment and destruction of those around him. They were facilitators of misery, so long as they hoped to make a profit. The *Diagnostic and Statistical Manual of Mental Disorders* (*DSM*) would deem them sociopathic – without conscience.

On 26 October 1972, our family convened a meeting. Dad was up from his eyrie in Spain. Mary was at school, but Mark and I were home for half-term. We were assembled in the lounge at Garden House. Dad wanted us to side with him and authorise borrowing more money. Auntie Jean and Mum were strongly opposed, and were finally making their stand.

Dad had recently passed his forty-seventh birthday and was looking quite trim. His weight used to oscillate, and he burned up more energy when he was manic, so his svelte profile was not a good sign. He strode up and down in front of the fireplace, laying out his case for more money, talking most of the time to the moulding that ran around the ceiling, with occasional demands made directly to each of us. He knew that the only way through to Mum and Auntie Jean was through his children, so he had been lobbying us with letters. Mark and I had heard it all before. We never discussed it between ourselves, though we had separately come to the same conclusion.

'I do hope the children were not too distressed,' Jean said afterwards to Mum. 'Of course, it was not a happy occasion, but I thought they both behaved extremely well under the circumstances.' It is odd to think of us as children in this situation, yet we certainly were: I was just thirteen.

Mark, fifteen, the scientist, was having none of Dad's nebulous plans. He argued that Dad was merely gambling on genetics, a subject that he thought his father did not understand very well. I was the one who took Dad to task on his numbers. By now, in addition to the other borrowing, I knew that the AMC mortgage alone was £250,000 for twenty-five years at 16 per cent. 16 per cent! I had just been given a fancy calculator, so it was a matter of using the compound-interest formula that I found in a maths book and plugging in numbers. If you did not pay off the interest, at the end of twenty-five years you would owe £10,218,560. Even if you paid the interest as you went along, you would pay five times as much as you borrowed – a million pounds on top of the original sum. We both told Dad flat out that we opposed borrowing any more money.

It got very ugly. Everyone was against him. Since he was losing the battle, he lashed out: he blamed our stupid attitudes on Mum, proclaiming – in a moment that left me aghast – that she was not fit to be our parent and he would evict her from the family home.

'I agree that I have neither the time nor the inclination to look after the children myself,' he said when Auntie Jean challenged him. 'I mean, I shall install a caretaker for the stud, you see, and I suppose I will have to find a housekeeper for them.'

By now I knew that when Dad started overusing his two signature pause phrases ('I mean' and 'you see'), it meant he was briefly lost for words. If he did not know what to do, I certainly did not. I started crying. If my friends at school had seen me blubbing – a teenager – I would have been humiliated. Dad had breached my carapace.

'I'm not . . . going to stay . . . on the stud . . . if that's how it's going to be!' I managed to blurt out. 'If Mum is going somewhere else, then I am going with her.'

'I gather Dick was extremely depressed,' Auntie Jean later said to Mum, 'and I must say I am not surprised; it was a far from uplifting session. I don't think for a moment that he will ask you to leave the house, though it is perfectly true that a stud manager is desperately needed.'

Mum wrote to Mark and Mary, but not to me, about the ongoing divorce. I suppose she thought me too young, and perhaps I was. The effect of Mum trying to protect me was that I heard Dad's version of events in daily letters, but I did not know for a long time that he was describing a world that none of the rest of us inhabited.

Auntie Jean wanted out of the stud all the more now, as it was causing her nothing but misery; this would leave Mum by herself. Mum was willing to do this only if Dad was out as well. So they began their torturous negotiations. Mary's half-term came a week after ours, which was unfortunate for her, since her experience was even worse.

'I was back for what I call my go-between days,' Mary told me. (We had both just read L. P. Hartley's book.) 'Nobody would talk to each other. They all talked to me. They were negotiating for the separation of Dad's new company, International Bloodstock Ltd, and Cheveley Park Stud. According to Dad, at least, I was meant to be convincing the others that what he wanted was the only thing that was possible. It was absurd that they could not talk to each other, yet it was totally understandable in retrospect, after all the talking they had done.'

That month, £54,000 was due in interest alone. In order to leave, Dad originally said he wanted a total value of £225,000 in horses, and for the loans to go with the stud. Though Dad had claimed that Forlorn River was worth a million pounds just a few months before, to achieve his purpose he now valued the horse at a tenth of that. If this seemed an unreasonable starting position, when all the muck had been shovelled to one side, Dad's new company somehow ended up with horses and stallion shares worth more than his original demand – £278, 950 – while only £73,200 of assets remained with the stud. It was a bit like a public–private partnership: Mum nationalised Dad's debt as her burden, and privatised the liquid assets allowing him to take them away to sell.

This dreadful business decision had one propulsion: the need to get Dad out. Mum was now primarily responsible for the desperate task of keeping Dad's inheritance alive. The odds against her were impossible, though I was shielded from the real world myself.

8

Paying for Torture Techniques in Private School

> Then took the other, as just as fair,
> And having perhaps the better claim,
> Because it was grassy and wanted wear.
>
> Robert Frost, 'The Road Not Taken'

It was 1974 and I had now moved on to Radley College, near Oxford. I was moaning about how little Nescafé Mum had given me. As she spooned it into a tin, showing me that I had enough for two cups a day all term, I thought she was just trying to teach me to be careful with money. It struck me as unworthy parsimony. I had no idea of the difficulty she was in – she had written to Auntie Jean describing a diet of little but eggs from the stud chickens, as she saved everything else for her children so we would be cushioned from the sudden change in circumstances.

Mum eventually had her divorce solicitor, the long-suffering Rosemary Sands, issue a demand to Dad for help with the school fees. I read his responsive tirade, as he sent a copy to each of us. He began by noting that he had £100 in the world, and he owed £6,000 on his overdraft on the Cambridge house on Clarendon Street. In other words, he was at minus £5,900. Dad was always talking about money in grandiose terms – and it was confusing to read that he was skint, since I was under the impression that he owned more than a hundred racehorses. Either he was being dishonest to the court and to his family, or he had blown £250,000 in a few months.

'The fundamental question at this point in time and as far as

I am concerned is whether there is any moral obligation or factual necessity for me to devote earning capacity to produce income for my ex-wife and the children,' he began. 'Clearly I could do this but it would be at the expense of fulfilling other obligations which I regard as being more urgent and of greater pressure on my conscience.'

I was left to speculate where I ranked in the universe.

'As far as the children are concerned, they have had an inordinate amount of money, time and thought spent on their upbringing and, as an educational consultant,' he continued, inventing his latest expertise, 'I would say they are just about achieving par.'

This was pretty dispiriting, and I had no idea what we would have to do to shoot a birdie or an eagle. Mark would soon become senior prefect at Radley, and Mary would later be appointed head girl in her final year of school. I don't think any of us had, at that point, ever taken a public exam without getting an A grade. We were all swots, though I looked on Mark as the true academic among us.

'Clive is the one who is suffering most from the claustrophobic attention of his mother and he may suffer for the rest of his life from the selfish attitudes and immaturity forced on him by such parental behaviour,' he concluded. I had no idea what he meant. I rarely even saw my mother, as I was at school for two-thirds of the year.

'Dick has this ability to make one feel in the wrong all the time,' Mum explained to Rosemary Sands. 'I suppose the principle of sending them to boarding school speaks for itself. Many people would criticise me as a neglectful mother for that precise reason.'

Meanwhile, Dad vanished off to Spain, sending illegible edicts from time to time about the state of the world and my own rather inadequate role within it.

At Radley, there was a local dialect – mostly novel terms for the class system that cascaded from the 'warden' to the 'social' master to the 'dons' to the 'senior prefect' to the lower forms of life. There were also divisions among family members: Mark was Stafford Smith MA (for 'major') and I was Stafford Smith MI ('minor'). At least there was no third brother, who would have been 'minimus'.

I was a 'stig' – a term from Clive King's 1963 book *Stig of the Dump*. It was not meant kindly. The main character of the book, Barney, goes exploring on the Downs near his grandparents' house, and tumbles into an old chalk pit where he meets Stig, who is some kind of caveman rummaging among the rubbish. The best Stig can manage is the occasional grunt, peering out from his den. The new boys were therefore Neanderthal neonates who had yet to learn the basics of public school life.

During my first few weeks, I was waterboarded. That was the kind of thing the boys did to each other, funded by the expensive school fees. I was on a scholarship, so I suppose I got it more or less for free. In the middle of Long Dormitory – two rows of thirty-six cubicles, either side of a wide walkway, in a cavernous space almost a hundred yards long – a dozen well-worn stairs led down to the bathroom. There were three or four toilets, and a series of baths. Between each bath was a slatted wooden duckboard.

The slightly older sociopaths would put a stig in the bath, slam the duckboard down on top and turn on the cold tap. If they were feeling particularly imaginative, when the young boy tried to poke his nose between the slats to breathe, they might use a pin to prick him. It is a strange bond I later had with some of the prisoners I met in Guantánamo Bay.

Thirty years after my Radley experience, I began one of my perverse hobbies, which was to research the antecedents of what the Bush administration blithely termed 'enhanced interrogation techniques'. Although neither George W. Bush nor (later) Donald J. Trump believed that waterboarding qualified as torture, the Spanish Inquisition had called it *tormento del agua* (water torture). Ironically, the Gestapo called it *verschärfte Vernehmung*, which translates as 'enhanced interrogation'.

As with most boarding schools, Radley was regimented like a detention centre. Dennis Silk was the Warden – the headmaster – and like in prison there was a code of honour. If you knew who had committed the crime, there was no sneaking on other boys, even if they were indulging in Gestapo-style torture.

'The privately educated Englishman . . . is the greatest dissembler on Earth,' says the fictional spy George Smiley in *The Secret Pilgrim* by John le Carré. 'Was, is now and ever shall be for as long as our disgraceful school system remains intact. Nobody will charm you so glibly, disguise his feelings from you better, cover his tracks more skilfully or find it harder to confess to you that he's been a damned fool.' It was the ultimate sin to rat, so we cannot be surprised at Boris Johnson's reaction when Priti Patel was found to have bullied her staff: far from demanding her resignation, he called for Conservatives to 'form a square round the Pritster'.

Boarding School Syndrome, and Post-Traumatic Stress Disorder (PTSD) from waterboarding, were only two of my brushes with 'mental illness' in school. I also suffered from anorexia. Around the age of sixteen I became body-obsessed, both because my mother and sister were constantly talking about diets and also due to my determination to turn my unprepossessing body into the physique of an England opening bowler (or at least play for Radley). I was up in the dark at 5 a.m. every day to splosh down in the rain to the gym to lift weights, which I complemented unwisely by counting every calorie and vomiting up even some of that. I was already my current height (6'3"), but I hovered under nine stone – six stone under my current weight. (I am not sure where it had gone, since there is still very little fat or muscle.)

Radley was not much interested in eating disorders, and

nobody noticed. From the start there was a highway with one destination: Oxbridge. Dad wanted me to get into his old college at Cambridge. 'I was feeling great this morning and I was hardly out of bed when a message came that Dad had rung asking me to call,' I once wrote to Mum. 'This I did. It was about the possibility of my getting into Corpus Christi College, which was all very thoughtful. However, when I mentioned that the work was quite hard, Dad suggested I'd find it much easier if I got up at 5 a.m. and do some work before I go to the gym.'

I had been strongly pressed by the school to do physics, chemistry, maths and further maths for A level, even though I wanted to be a writer, not a scientist. But I finally began to find the courage to rebel. I had finally got into the First XI at cricket and had just won my colours. The physics S-level paper was scheduled for the same day as our cricket match against the Young Australians. I begged to be allowed to take the paper at another time, either before or after the match, so I could play. But that was not the way the system was aligned. The exam was in the gym and I just sat there glumly, pondering what this meant. The magnets of life were set either side of me: a guilty pull from my indoctrination, against the tug of the revelation that I was a slave to a future I did not want. I had to make a complete break. I did not write anything at all. It was the first exam I had ever failed, and I failed it with conviction.

I may have been a rebel in Oxbridge terms, but I was still more Henry Tudor than Karl Marx. At that moment, an opportunity arrived to apply to the University of North Carolina in Chapel Hill, on a scholarship endowed by John Motley Morehead, the founder of the chemical corporation Union Carbide. His stipulation was that only young men could apply, and they had to come from one of England's top-ten private schools. I had never heard of Chapel Hill, I had no idea where North Carolina was, but for me at least it was the key to the prison gates.

★

I look at my contribution to the life of Radley College as one of my own failures. When my brother was senior prefect he worked to make some changes, abolishing the routines of 'fagging', where the older boys could force the stigs to do menial chores for them and even had the right to beat them. As head boy, my only legacy was to raise the weekend beer limit allowed in the Senior Common Room by half a pint.

There were much larger issues facing education than this. In the US I would later learn a great deal about an enforceable right to equality. One case that struck me in particular was *Tennessee Small Schools Systems* v. *McWherter*, which involved state education. Because much of the funding for schools came from the local tax base, a neighbourhood full of rich white families tended to receive a disproportionately large education budget compared to an area populated by less-advantaged parents. The judges noted that spending per pupil varied by more than 100 per cent, from $1,823 to $3,669, depending on the county.

This obviously meant that if you were born with a silver spoon in your mouth, it would metamorphose into gold, while wooden spoons developed woodworm. The Bill of Rights provides that no state shall 'deny to any person within its jurisdiction the equal protection of the laws'. The state was providing very unequal protection, and the Tennessee Supreme Court ordered that it should be evened out.

In the UK, matters are far worse. Spending per state student has dropped significantly since the last Labour government and was, as of 2018, £4,600 where my son attends school. Compare this to Radley College, the 'public school' where I went (set in eight hundred acres and with a private golf course) – the annual fees are £40,125 at the time of writing, although the various clubs and opportunities cost extra (close to £1,000 for music lessons alone), and on top of that the school boasts an additional £3.28 million a year from its charitable fund. This means that the students have ten times as much spent on them per capita as do state students.

Private education threatens the integrity of the entire society. In common with many private schools, Radley gave me a very privileged, academic education that had little to do with the world outside our carefully manicured grounds. Meanwhile, among the British judges who condemn the prisoners before them (most of whom come from less-advantaged backgrounds), 74 per cent are from private schools. We think we are making progress, as this has dropped from 76 per cent in the past thirty years.

After observing them for many years, I am not convinced that this cadre of judges has much insight into the reasons why people end up committing the 'crimes' we deem worthy of prison – and nor do they have any more insight into the impact their education has had on them than I did.

9

Dad Dabbles in Normal Life and Finds It Wanting

[He] was, like a good salesman, an optimist. Salesmen, whose
primary characteristic and main asset is their ability to keep
selling, constantly recast the world in positive terms. Discour-
agement for everyone else is merely the need to improve reality
for them.

Michael Wolff on Donald J. Trump, *Fire and Fury*

On 31 August 1977, Dad was declared bankrupt based on the
petition of a credit card company. The court amalgamated
the case with his other debts. The receiver sought to 'commit
the bankrupt' for his failure to file a 'statement of affairs' detailing his finances. Presumably this would once have put Dad in
debtors' prison, a practice much abused by Mad King George
in the eighteenth century.

Poetry, as close a proxy for emotion as perhaps Dad had, was
one indicator of his mood. Now Dad wrote:

These trees are still, and yet the West Wind's strong –
Beyond the bay the clouds scud o'er the hill.
The waves are white-tipped, foaming, lithe and long
The world's in motion, yet those trees are still.
This place is calm and yet the world's at war;
No peace of mind – all trouble and alarm.
The motive of man's life is 'more and more'
And chaos reigns – and yet this place is calm.
These trees are still – and while they stay that way
Hope lingers on that we may banish strife.

The ripples in this calm may steal away
And win men's souls at last for love and life.

By now I was set on escape to America, and it was possible
for me to put Dad to one side and forget him altogether, save
for an epistle from him once or twice a week. So I did just that.
His frequent letters described, in vague terms, a new company
he wished to establish called Equus. He never acknowledged
that he had pinched the name from Peter Shaffer's 1973 play, in
which psychiatrist Martin Dysart treats seventeen-year-old
Alan Strang, who had bizarrely blinded six horses. The story
was inspired by a real-life incident that happened in Suffolk,
not far from Cheveley Park Stud.

In the play, Strang holds the animals as god-figures, and he
thinks he has betrayed them by allowing a young woman, Jill,
to seduce him in the stables. Dysart, disillusioned with his job,
knows that if he 'cures' the boy, all he has to offer is a return to
a dull, normal life that lacks passion. Perhaps, Dysart ponders,
reducing someone to a meaningless existence is no cure at all.

Dad was facing up to his greatest fear: 'normal' life.

His lover, Dawn, was now his second wife, and she insisted that
she would not live with him if he did not provide financial support. Dad's mood did come down far enough for him to
experiment with the kind of normalcy that left Dr Dysart so
sceptical. He returned to England, promising Dawn he would
provide for my infant half-sister, Katie, by working as a salesman for Saxonfoam, a manufacturer of home insulation. When
he began in October 1979, his first week's pay was £38.92, but
within four months he was bringing in more than £2,000 a
month in commissions – a good salary for 1980.

For a while, Saxonfoam fitted Dad-the-Salesman. He convinced himself that the product helped to reduce fuel waste,
which – with two scientists in the family, Mark and Mary, both

of whom were increasingly devoted to the issue of climate change – allowed him to see his work in the grand perspective. He rapidly became the leading Saxonfoam salesman, setting records and earning the respect of his colleagues. He even started trying to buy a house for his second family. No bank was going to put up money for an undischarged bankrupt, so Dad began selling his sister Jean on backing 'Katie's Cottage'.

Unfortunately, the tide turned once more, as it did with every moon. Dad could see various opportunities for Saxonfoam. If you were selling insulation, why not include double glazing? All this required was a joint project with a glazing company, and Dad picked Cunningham Glass. A heat pump would also reduce the cost of warming the home, so that was an obvious move. If the customer could not afford it, Dad suggested a deal with a mortgage company who could raise the cash. Saxonfoam were not particularly happy about him selling the products of other companies, but short of firing him there was not a lot they could do about it.

Yet he was only coming out of the starting blocks: comfort was one matter, but everyone should, he thought, aspire to leisured luxury. Dad began advising his clients on the installation of cheap swimming pools. Then he wondered why they would want to be in England during the nine months of the year when no sane person would want to swim there. How about his beloved Spain? Dad offered to help them buy their dream home on the Costa del Sol.

By now, the management at Saxonfoam were very concerned. Dad discussed his ideas with Jack Lever, who was theoretically his manager, though Dad was beginning to see the relationship the other way around.

'As I see it, my marketing plan is exactly in line with Saxonfoam's interests, you see,' he explained. 'I mean, the logic is obvious. The most expensive and difficult part of the marketing operation is obtaining the lead, getting the confidence of the customer and closing the sale. You know that. And yet having spent all that money and gone to all that trouble, Saxonfoam says goodbye.'

Lever nodded dubiously.

'I have in mind all kinds of things, you see,' Dad went on. 'Central heating, replacement windows, solar heating, swimming pools, tennis courts, kitchen and bathroom fittings, and any other products we can think of. What do you say?'

'Let me give it some thought,' said Lever. Dad's idea might be fine in theory, but Saxonfoam was a small company trying to move forward gradually. 'Gradual' was not a gear at which Dad wanted his world to operate. But Lever was facing an increasing number of complaints. Dad was not just encouraging all the other sales staff to join in with him, he was bubbling up with outrage when customers did not accept his judgement.

The day after Valentine's Day 1981, a Sunday, Mary dropped in to see how Dad, Dawn and Kate were in the home they rented near Farnham. Dad was out. Kate was playing, and Mary went up to where Dawn was resting. They sat on the bed talking. Dad was escalating rapidly. The night before, he had shouted at Auntie Jean on the phone, leaving his sister in floods of tears. Surreptitiously, preparing for what she now feared was the inevitable divorce, Dawn had taped that conversation, and she played it back to Mary. They also reviewed two letters Dad had written to potential Saxonfoam clients, his vitriol spilling off the typewriter ribbon.

'Later that evening . . . I kept feeling it cannot be so,' Mary remembered. 'The appallingness of the letters kept coming back . . . proof that it was happening.'

Four days later, Dad rang Mary to tell her Dawn had left. 'We had a slight disagreement, and during the course of it I am afraid that I was forced to give her a "little slap". She just would not listen, you see. I mean, she was just unbalanced.' He could not believe that Dawn had deserted him when the pressure of work was so severe. 'I mean, she has been beastly over the last four weeks. How can I keep up my work rate if there is nobody there to cook meals?'

That evening, Mary went back to Farnham. Dad was speaking to one of his colleagues at Saxonfoam on the phone, and when he hung up he asked her what she thought – had he been rude? She thought he had been extremely aggressive, which was not uncharacteristic, but she settled for suggesting that he could have handled it more diplomatically. As was his wont, Dad was on and off the phone all evening, but he made an effort to be particularly polite. In the meantime, though, he would hear nothing in Dawn's favour and was intent on building his empire. He had plans for the massive expansion of Saxonfoam, and promised to make at least a quarter of a million in the next six months with his ideas.

Dad was not recognising reality at all. Dawn had not left him, he insisted, because he had hit her. She had left, he said, because his sister Jean and her worthless husband Bob had failed to help him buy a family home, Katie's Cottage. It was all their fault.

Reviewing Dad's life, I came across plenty of people who thought him a fraud, and a smaller number who were very compassionate. Jack Lever fell into the second category, and his efforts brought to mind John Mills at Cambridge almost twenty years before. Lever had just finished calming down another angry customer when he asked for a meeting with Dad.

'Over the last week or so I know you have been making very strenuous efforts to further and protect the reputation of both Saxonfoam and yourself,' he began, choosing his words carefully. 'Unfortunately, these efforts are resulting in an increasing amount of adverse return. The harder and longer you work at a "problem" the more adverse the reaction. This would never have happened with the "old" Dick Stafford Smith and I am sure we would all very much like to see the old Dick Stafford Smith back again!'

He told Dad to take a holiday. 'Total relaxation starting now as you walk out of the office, not in a week's time.' He said that Dad's colleagues all liked him, but felt the same way – he had just been overdoing it.

He went on to say that they would continue to pay Dad based on his average income over the past three months, even though he would not be working, as he was a valued and exceptional salesman. 'I've got to stress that in return for this retainer, we expect you not to lift so much as a finger . . . much less a telephone receiver or pen . . . or to get involved in anything that remotely resembles "work".'

Lever would welcome Dad back in two weeks, rested, fully refreshed and running smoothly in top gear – but not roaring along at 60,000 revs per minute as he had been of late, the engine boiling over. 'Listen to your friends, Dick,' he concluded. 'Now is the moment to take a little time to wind down.'

I was not sure how Dad would respond to this, but it was all kindly said, kindly meant.

Mary decided she had to try to get Dad to see a doctor. She knew it was going to be an unpleasant battle, no matter how she approached it, but he was her dad, and she felt she had no option. She, like Dawn, had been preparing for an inevitable future, so she had kept comprehensive notes of their conversations. She suggested he might be overwrought.

'You're not going to start that again, are you?' he demanded. 'You have already caused huge problems saying that in the past. I've told you, don't ever – repeat, *ever* – accept vicarious evidence!' Dawn was the problem, not him.

Mary pointed out that she was not relying on hearsay, but what she saw before her. She continued gently to suggest he had stressed himself and should at least get a check-up.

'OK, then,' Dad relented. 'If you decide . . . on careful reflection . . . that you are right, then go and see Dr McCleod and arrange a meeting for me to see her friend.' He could not bring himself to say 'psychiatrist'. 'If you decide you are very wrong then say you are sorry to your dear old dad who has the most to forgive – or should it be the other way round? I am not sure. Maybe I'm the one who has done the rotten job in bringing up such a useless, unthinking, stupid, ill-mannered, humourless daughter-of-the-devil.'

Dad decided to take up Lever's offer. Spain was always his nirvana and the next day he was about to get on the plane when he called Mary. 'I spoke to Dr McCleod earlier this evening,' he said, from Luton Airport. 'I've been up all night and am a bit disorientated. She said she would show my letters to the head shrinker, and see if she wants to see you, me, us, Clive, Auntie Jean, your ma, or good old Uncle Tom Cobbly.'

As background for the doctor who, she hoped, would be the first to evaluate Dad since 1965, Mary wrote a stream of consciousness:

Verbal bully. Unpredictable in behaviour with other people – can be extremely embarrassing. Hypercritical – with unfair criticism. Either in a deep depression or hypermanic. Unsocial working hours. On the phone constantly – disregard for money, telephone bill. Erratic. Raising unrealistic hopes – constant exaggeration. Distrust. Lying by omission. Violence. Irresponsible. Verbal diarrhoea. Enthusiasm. Dogmatic about his own talents and virtues. Believes absolutely that the ends justify the means. This is fundamental to his cruelty. Hit Mum once, burst her eardrum. Hit Granny Smith – she hit him back. Finds your weak spot and then hammers at it. Makes you feel total weariness, both mentally and physically. Creates distrust between friends. People around him always on trial.

At the end, Mary wrote a note to herself for when she hoped to meet with the doctors: 'Make all points and multiply by ten or so!'

There is a great deal in Mary's notes that definitely happened, though I did not agree with some of her conclusions. But then I wouldn't, would I? Mary would see me through the same lens much of the time – as it was clearer to her than to me that I was our father's son. Though I could see this intellectually – I had picked up some of his mannerisms – it was still rather difficult to be told I was behaving like Dad when I would get into a loud argument with someone. At one level, though, to be compared to him gave me a sense of empathy. For example, I don't think that Dad consciously lied to anyone: he was trying to persuade them to what he thought was an obvious truth. I don't think he meant to be cruel: he truly thought that if the goal was marvellous, then people were foolish not to try and reach it. He strongly believed that all his Saxonfoam clients should be encouraged to enjoy themselves in their Spanish swimming pools, and it is difficult to see this as morally wrong.

Mary thought that he was unrealistic, and there she was probably correct. Dad did not want to inhabit the real world.

For two weeks on the Costa del Sol, he relaxed a little and thought a great deal. Unfortunately, the more he lay in the bath, the more certain he was that he was correct – both about the future of Saxonfoam and on the broader question of who was rational and who was not. On his arrival back at Luton, he announced that he was not willing to meet with a psychiatrist unless it was to get Mary or Dawn the help they so obviously needed. Dr McCleod told a dispirited Mary that while it seemed clear he needed help, he could not be forced.

I wondered what it took to force someone. The classic rule is that someone can only be sectioned if they are a danger to themselves or others. We tend to think of that in terms of physical danger but – even if we were to deem his 'little slap' insufficient – Dad was in danger of destroying what he had left in life. Short of involuntary commitment, he had to be convinced that help was in his best interests, and for that it would be important to eliminate the stigma of 'mental illness' in society and, most important, in himself.

Dad was met on his return by a lengthy missive from Mum: 'I am going to make just one effort to write an objective letter to you which I hope you will kindly read through, perhaps even twice, and please take the meaning of it as a whole; don't batten onto one or two phrases out of context to shoot the whole thing down on those. You can decide before you read it that it is illogical, because I am a woman, but that won't affect the sense of it.'

I can imagine her at her typewriter in the house she had bought in Fordham, where she had spent so much of her youth. She would probably have prepared for the task with a watered glass of Scotch; this evening would justify a successor. She was a speedy typist, so her thoughts would have transmitted fluidly to the keys.

'First, the facts. You accept you are manic-depressive.' It was a strong opening gambit. Dad rarely accepted this, and then only as a wonderfully positive temperament that allowed him to do so much work. 'This involves three periods or moods in a series: depressed and low, middling, and hyperactive. These repeat themselves in cycles, to a greater or lesser extent. To take the middle "mood" first, this is the time when you live a reasonably settled life, when you build up carefully and consistently some plan or opportunity (e.g. the good work you did in estate management, building up the stud, managing Caius College property, building a reputation and establishing a clientele with Saxonfoam, etc.). Perhaps not wildly exciting, but successful and satisfying to a point, and reassuring to those who live around you.'

This would make sense to many, of course, but it would not appeal to Dad. Indeed, I tend towards his point of view: for me the idea of a nine-to-five job is a slow descent into the Lethe. I respect people who do such work and I think they should be paid much more than me, since I get much more pleasure out of my job than most. But the idea of having to do the same thing eight hours a day, five days a week, fifty weeks a year, for fifty years – in total, for *one hundred thousand hours* . . . I have dabbled in it, and it is my nightmare too.

She was not going to win the debate with this line.

'On one side of this mood we have the depressed state,' Mum continued. 'At this time you can hardly see how to get through the next twenty-four hours. You see everything in the blackest possible light and those around you must constantly encourage you, and point out what is obvious to them – that as night follows day, you are shortly going to be on the up again.'

This was the black dog that Dad wanted desperately to avoid. I am fortunate that though I am much like Dad at the more manic end of the spectrum, I have thankfully never experienced the depressed end. It is surely the aspect of his trifecta that everyone would agree should be treated and, if possible, eliminated.

Then she came to the present: 'At the other end of the extreme, we have the hyperactive mood. At this stage you start up the most brilliant and imaginative schemes but even you must have noticed by now that *none* of these comes to anything: the Cambridge plan, new towns for Spain, Parknasilla's golf course, horse training in Holland, Equus, and a host of other projects.' She could have listed another ten that were now no more than fading typewriter ribbon, and she dared not mention the stud. Even this brief list was a terrible epitaph: everything he had ever done was a failure. True or false, it would crush Dad to see himself this way.

Unfortunately, it was true. Mum knew it. I knew it. Everyone around him knew it.

'Now why is this? Every one of these aborted schemes has come to an end with a row. Every time supposedly someone else has let you down. You have had the idea, you have worked hard to get people interested, then when it looks as if at last this one will get off the ground, you put them under so much pressure that somehow you break the scheme. You go on to something new. It is as if the responsibility of being successful is too much and when the moment comes to consolidate the launching of a scheme, you run away, and it is left as nothing without your driving force.'

Again, I disagreed with Mum about some of the details. It seemed to me that while the pattern was always the same, the path to inevitable dissolution was slightly different. Dad would be manic, he would have an idea, and he would think it so exceptional that he would want to see it in action today. He would enthuse others, yet he simply could not handle the slow pace of the world that others inhabited. He would be working twenty hours in every twenty-four, while the rest of the world was nine-to-five. Dad's 'work' never involved making the business operate in any functional sense, but rather cajoling others to act – the role of the eternal salesman. For all his insistence that he was an 'implementation planner', Dad was a dreadful manager and needed someone to translate his ideas into practice. Perhaps the reason Dad's management of the stud had been reasonably successful for a few years was that Mum had been the one to make sure everything happened when it should. No project after the stud ever actually crashed; none of them even got off the ground.

Looking at this, I can see myself reflected in the mirror. I do not pretend that I am an 'implementation' expert. I have had people around me, over many years, who have helped translate my own ideas into a reality, whether dealing with a death penalty case in Louisiana or a drone assassination in Waziristan. One of the charities I founded – Reprieve – boasts that it is a limber organisation that leaps at the latest human rights abuse, rather than spending months debating which is the best path to take. For many years, most of those leaps were based on my sudden obsession with an issue. None would have gone as far if others had not carried them forward.

On the other hand, from time to time I have been criticised for leaping suddenly off the ship without even a lifebelt, when the idea was unrealistic. By and large, again I beg to differ. They were not bad ideas; the simple truth is that they went nowhere as, standing alone, I could not make them happen. (One of many examples is when I decided that we should take on police corruption in New Orleans. It was a worthy goal – after all, one police officer told me that he was going down to court to testi-lie rather than testify. I had many ideas about how we could confront this, such as the monthly 'Stop the PIG' award – PIG standing for 'perjury in government'. But I was so keen to rush ahead that I failed to bring the other members of the office along, so it went nowhere – and the police continued to lie.)

I wondered whether Dad would have got on better if he had always had someone steady but brilliant (like my mother) willing to help carry an idea forward. Or perhaps he should have been encouraged to follow a different path, where he would not have needed such a facilitator to the same degree. Why tell a manic person that he should be a factory inspector (too dull for him) or gamble on the racing industry (alluring to him, but far too uncertain)? Dad's temperament was much better suited to the creative arts than it was to business.

Mum signed her letter 'with love', and she really meant it. She wanted nothing more than for Dad to be happy and to succeed. I wondered what was gushing through his mind as he read her letter.

Dad's life was strewn all around, but he had spent two weeks in Malaga piecing together a jigsaw that made sense to him.

His second wife had left him, taking their daughter – but he had only given Dawn that 'little slap' because she was 'unbalanced'. Saxonfoam had paid him to go on holiday for two weeks to try to regain his own balance, but Jack Lever had it wrong: Dad had thought through his plans for the expansion of the business, and they were good . . . no, they were exceptional.

His daughter Mary had been trying to get him to see a psychiatrist, and even though she was a scientist, she was still a woman, and therefore probably could not see true logic. His ex-wife had just sent him a long screed that illustrated how she was trapped in her middle-class, middle-of-the-dull-road life, walking blindly past the extraordinary.

The mind is a machine for making itself right, and Dad's machine was highly tuned.

'What more can I say than "thank you" for spending so much time and thought on a subject which hardly deserves it,' Dad began in his reply to Mum, with a false modesty that inevitably presaged what was to come. 'Your analysis and diagnosis is extremely acute and in ninety-nine cases out of a hundred, and possibly even 999,999 out of a million your proposed treatment would be right – and that's not a bad ratio of success. Unfortunately, it is not right in this case . . . and in making that claim I do so in all humility but in absolute certainty. I was given a set of talents which are very unusual and in some ways extremely frightening. This is a statement of "no pride" since talents are either genetically or God-given (or both!) and personal pride is only to be taken in their use not in their origin.'

Any expert reading his opening salvo would immediately be reaching for the manual to check the various ways in which grandiosity might contribute to a diagnosis.

'My set of talents are not quite unique since Clive has almost exactly the same set,' he pointed out. 'Doubtless there are others with similar sets that have been crippled by the world around them before they are allowed to develop.'

I weighed his words when I read them years later. I knew he viewed me – as I sometimes saw myself – as my father's son. His normal pattern, though, was to add in what a useless person I was, and detail how my supposed genius had been stamped out by various small-minded teachers. On the other hand, to be dubbed his true heir was perhaps even more worrying.

'It has taken me a long time to understand my talents, and be able to control them and the frustrations which the environment imposes on them,' he said. 'I think, hope and trust that you will see some difference this time around! I am living and working on my own since it is clear that no one can cope with me in a hard-working, hard-living mood. I am earning money as well as dreaming dreams.'

Dreaming his dreams at Saxonfoam, Dad was never going to be satisfied peddling insulation, any more than it would satisfy me. He wanted to turn the company into some kind of multinational that could bring leisured happiness to millions, and perhaps end the threat to the world's climate along the way.

'I am even implementing my plans since it appears that I am not only the best planner around but I am also the best "implementor" [sic], the best salesman, etc. And a most modest fellow to boot!' He was trying to be amusing here, but Mum would not have read it that way. She knew that implementation – as well as spelling – was among his flaws.

Dad still had two decades to live, but it seemed increasingly as if the catastrophe would continue – with none of his ideas going anywhere while he became increasingly divorced from everyone around him.

10

Millard Farmer Tilts at Legal Windmills

Was off jes' now, some place in the Past
Country-back roads an' men cuttin' grass;
Swelterin' days an' endless nights;
Bloodhound dogs an' shotgun shells.
Back to the Chain Gang in 'seventy-one . . .
Long time ago, a diff'rent world!
Glad I ain't there no more.
But I go off recollectin' the Time
When I was in the Chain Gang
An' that was my life.

Jack Howard Potts, 'Under Death Sentence'

I went to the University of North Carolina, intending to study journalism. During the first summer vacation I had to do an internship with the police, as part of the scholarship founder's vision that we should learn to respect the voices of authority. I was dispatched to the Los Angeles County Sheriff's Department (LASD), and it was educational in all kinds of ways, most of them unintended (as was my relationship with Dad). First, a sergeant demonstrated how a polygraph worked, and how to cheat when lying. He hooked me up to the various sensors that were meant to read your emotions and identify a falsehood. With each suspect he had to calibrate the machine, for which he would ask various anodyne questions. During this process, he instructed me to think the most erotic thoughts I could; this would, he said, tune the machine at that level. Then, when the examiner approached the inculpatory areas, he said I should continue to focus on erotica and lie however I liked. I lied and passed with ease. My only problem was keeping up the sexual fantasies: I could do it readily enough when he asked if my birthday was 9 July, but found it challenging when he asked me to confirm my mother's maiden name.

I witnessed my first murder in LA. One evening I was with eight cops in a diner where they were extorting free coffee and doughnuts from the owner. A call came in, and they all walked to their cars before driving to the scene, brushing other vehicles to the side of the road with their flashing blue lights. We encountered a skinny black man with a blade who was obviously out of his mind on drugs – it was the height of the angel dust epidemic. He was babbling incoherently, and stumbling, oblivious, towards eight service revolvers. I assumed the cops would issue a loud warning, and then maybe use a nightstick on him if that did not work. I was wrong. They did shout at him to put the knife down, but when he ignored them, they killed him right in front of me. It was an era before mobile phones with cameras, and I suspect that it was not the only unjustified police shooting that month. I was sickened. I wrote to Sheriff Peter J. Pitchess offering to appear at an inquest, but I never heard back.

This pushed me towards a life I wanted to live. Soon after, I was in a bar after work with a Scottish guy who had somehow found his way into the LASD uniform. He had promised me something other than weak American lager. That is when he told me about Millard Farmer and Team Defense Project Inc. 'Bet you something,' he said. 'Bet you don't go work with him. You'll be off after them big bucks, you college types.'

My father had given me good cause to hate gambling, but this was one of the few bets I was willing to take.

I thanked the Morehead Foundation for LA, but I just wasn't willing to go on the planned experience the next summer, which was a business internship to learn about John Motley

Morehead's love of lucre. Instead I set up my own summer with this Millard Farmer.

Immediately after I arrived at the chaotic Team Defense headquarters in Atlanta, Kimellen Tunkle, the paralegal who ran the office, announced that we were driving to Mississippi to join a solidarity march with some people who were on strike at a chicken processing plant, just across the border from Alabama. It was a glorious summer day, and we set off in a hire car in party mood, Millard at the wheel alongside Kimellen, with me in the back with Lisa Ferdinand. I had an immediate, unassuageable crush on Lisa, as she was – and no doubt still is – wildly beautiful, on top of her compassionate politics. She seemed far above me, though, as she was working at Team Defense through VISTA (Volunteers in Service to America) – a brilliant project created by President Kennedy to fund young people who helped those beset by poverty.

I was excited about our destination as well. Mississippi was almost mythological for the dark days of the civil rights movement, taught as US history at UNC, but it was clearly still part of current affairs. The women – they were all women, mostly black women – on strike at the plant were complaining about their work conditions. The issue I remember most starkly was that they were only allowed to go unauthorised to the toilet twice a week while working, and otherwise had to wait for an official break – but this was merely one of the absurd rules to which they were subjected if they wanted their miserable pay packet. It was a company town where, after the abolition of slavery, the local people had to buy from the company store and would rack up such debts that they could never leave. The white man who owned the plant called it his 'plantation'. It was my first introduction to yellow dog laws – the state did not allow strikes, so the owner could bus in scabs from the neighbouring county, where plenty of people were short of work.

It was a day out for me, a stroll through a small Southern town with cottages set back behind white picket fences, and semi-tropical flowers in full bloom. We came level with an old lady, a stooped grandmother with an apron, who was regarding us through thick glasses over her garden gate. I wished her good afternoon with a smile.

'Go home, you nigger lovers!' she spat back. 'What business you got here?'

I recoiled. Then we encountered the counter-march that met us in the centre of the town. Almost all Southern town centres are similar, with a granite-grey stone courthouse of two or three storeys, perhaps shaded by an oak tree, invariably flanked by the memorial to the Confederacy. After the disaster of 1865 – when the South lost the Civil War – a compromise had been struck with the Reconstruction government: the soldiers in grey could be remembered, but their statues would have to stand with empty bandoliers, their rifles forever without ammunition. Such a stolid man stood eyeing us from one corner of the courthouse square, stone-dressed in his battlefield grey. On the other side, his heirs awaited: the massed ranks of the Ku Klux Klan, in their white uniforms, their wizard hats and veiled faces. Like the grandmother before them, they were making it very clear that we were unwelcome in their town.

A stand-off ensued. A few brave civil rights advocates bellowed their speeches, challenged by the shaken fists of the Klan. Meanwhile, Highway Patrol officers separated the two sides. They were themselves all white – it was 1980, and the civil rights laws had only just begun to filter down as far as Mississippi – and wearing reflective sunglasses, their allegiance uncertain if violence did break out.

This went on for an hour or more before we decided to hightail it back to Georgia. We had to return past the picket fences and cottages, now with their white lace curtains drawn, only the occasional stirring to betray the smouldering blue-rinse hair behind. When we got to our car, there was a clean bullet hole through the radiator – Kimellen was the one who had to explain that to the rental company. We headed home, less exuberant, unsure that our excursion had achieved much.

I was left to wonder at the people I had encountered. As a privileged white kid, I had been at Radley where slurs were tossed around with abandon. I was only just confronting how horribly wrong that had been. The Klan seemed a sorry lot to me, yet they were convinced they were genetically superior to all black people. If my father was deemed 'mentally ill', what about these people in their shocking white hoods? They were far less rational than Dad – and more of a threat to those around them.

I began to wonder whether a large slice of the world was mad, or whether it might make sense to look at everyone through a different lens.

The folk at Team Defense did not know what to do with me. I was twenty years old, I had never been to the South before, I knew nothing about the law and my naivety was unblemished. Kimellen thought at the very least I might be able to entertain the men on death row, and act as a go-between when a crisis arose. I was excited at being trusted with a task of my own; my only reservation was the loss of Lisa's radiant smile welcoming me into the office each morning. The focus was to be on Jack Potts, who was taking up much of Millard Farmer's time. Having found himself on death row, with nobody who gave a damn, Jack would get depressed and decide he might as well end it all. He would try to forgo any challenge to his conviction and be executed, whereupon suddenly the small cadre of death penalty opponents were all around him trying to change his mind. Then he would decide that life had meaning after all, and therefore agree to continue with his appeals. Thus the cycle would repeat.

So I drove in my old V W Karmann Ghia down to Reidsville in Georgia to establish residence there. On the way I had to go through a series of towns, each of which was like the other in one respect: the speed limit gradually reduced from 55 to 50 to 45 to 40 to 35 to 30 over the space of a quarter-mile. I had been warned: the police generated a lot of income from speeding fines, and they would use each sign to trap you. With my out-of-state number plate, I slowed to 28 mph at the first sign.

Each town's other signage set out a different speciality. As I came into Vidalia, I was told that it was 'Home of the Sweet Onion'; Claxton was 'Home of the Fruit Cake', of which I became fond; when I eventually came to Reidsville, it was 'Home of the Georgia State Prison'.

I had arrived at death row. Ironically, I got there six years before Larry Lonchar; he was still graduating from different prisons up in Michigan. I had made it all the way from England to this odd backwater in rural Georgia. Not many people were looking to move to Reidsville – most wanted out, including almost a hundred condemned men.

My landlord was a local lawyer by the name of Wensley Hobby. I went to his office to hand over my summer rent of $150 a month. On the desk was a plastic clockwork mouse. When I asked what it was doing there, he beamed and dived in his pinstripe suit to the carpet with the mouse in hand, to demonstrate how it buzzed around the floor.

Everyone was odd in Reidsville – just as I was an alien to them. The metaphorical railway tracks divided white from black, and back then I did not have the courage to challenge the local mores, so my room was in a large, otherwise empty house in the white zone. I took a photograph of the pickup truck that was parked in front of my new home with the bumper sticker 'God, Guns & Guts Made America: Let's Keep All Three!' I had bought a mattress at a local charity shop, where the young woman at the cash register had just watched the movie *10* and had her hair done in tight cornrows like Bo Derek. I chatted with her, wondering what she thought of the fact that black women had been wearing their hair like that since the

Egyptians 5,000 years earlier. She seemed surprised when I suggested that her fancy new fashion statement was merely copying those from the other side of the tracks.

The Georgia State Prison was a short and sweaty drive out of town, through the pine trees. Initially, I found it intimidating. To visit the men on death row I had, first, to pass by the guards. Then I was ushered into a visiting area with a large rusting metal fan. Up in the tower was the chamber with its electric chair. Once a week the authorities tested the prison generator to make sure the chair was in fine fettle. All the lights dimmed.

I was not sure what I was meant to talk to the men about. My privileged background? My plan to pop home to England at the end of the summer? As it turned out, it was easy. Johnny Mack Westbrook, a mentally disabled man, was surprised to have a visitor at all. Although his family was vast, with more than a dozen siblings, he had seen nobody but Millard and Kimellen from outside the prison for six years. Even for me, a twenty-year-old, it was hard to see him as more than a child.

There was Billy Moore, a gentle Christian who had pled guilty to murder and been sentenced to death, although the family of the victim had forgiven him. An older man called Billy Birt gave me advice. 'Clive, don't you be taking no lip from those women folk,' he said one day in his almost incomprehensible drawl, his bright blue eyes sparkling. 'Mah mother-in-law gave me trouble one time, and I went around they-ar and burned her house down. Di'n't give me no more trouble after that.'

On 9 July, I celebrated my twenty-first birthday. Dad wrote to me. Somehow, far away in London, because he was earning nothing and unlikely to, his legal aid lawyer had worked out a deal where he paid only £4,500 on his many debts. 'On the whole I think we did quite well!' Dad wrote.

The same month, Troy Gregg, Timothy 'Wes' McCorquodale, Johnny Johnson and David Jarrell escaped from the prison. It was the first death row breakout in Georgia history. They dyed their prison outfits to look like correctional officer uniforms, made a few fake badges, sawed through their bars and walked out. An aunt had left a car in the visitors' parking lot. Less than thirty-six hours later, Troy was beaten to death by two of Wes's Hells Angels friends in North Carolina. Johnny later said Troy had been hitting on the 'ol' lady' of one of the bikers. Troy's body was found floating in a lake.

He had been a sorry figure, as he had given his name to the seminal case of *Gregg* v. *Georgia*, the 1976 Supreme Court decision that had effectively revalidated the death penalty in the US after its temporary abolition in 1972. Dying at the hands of the Hells Angels may have only spared him the electric chair. After three days of freedom, the others were flushed out with tear gas, and driven in chains back to Georgia.

Soon, I had to go back to university, where the academic discourse seemed slightly irrelevant. I entered into negotiations to avoid spending more time in class. An English teacher allowed me to do another rather grand project I had in mind – writing a book – in lieu of showing up for class for the first half of 1981. It was going to be called *Life on Death Row* and it would be a study of Jack Potts UDS ('under death sentence'). I figured the least I could do for Team Defense was to spend my last semester trying to keep Jack on an even keel.

I made arrangements to head back to Georgia.

My second tour of duty in the Deep South began with a swing through Louisiana and Mississippi accompanying Millard, soaking up his experience of a real world with which I was only passingly familiar. The three lawyers with Team Defense were essentially the only people willing to do death penalty work full-time in the Southern States, and they would range from Texas across to Florida. Millard and I listened to jazz at Jimmy's in New Orleans until three in the morning before driving seven hours up to Parchman, the Mississippi State Penitentiary, to visit four men on death row there.

Millard was my mentor. In many ways he was like Dad, though his contrariness was channelled more effectively: he had blown most of his own inheritance on helping indigent people get off death row, rather than gambling on horses. He could be rude and outrageous in his unyielding and barely comprehensible rural Georgia accent, but only when he was 'conflictioneering' – a term he coined for creating discord in the smooth-running railroad that was designed to take a prisoner to the electric chair. He hated the rigid court rules that set the schedule, and in his attempts to intimidate racist judges, he consistently strayed close to contempt of court.

Millard and I followed the road I would later come to know so well, up to Indianola and Cleveland; more small towns with railroad tracks dividing black from white, with the same small-town cops loitering under the pecan trees trying to pick people off to raise money from speeding tickets. Millard – dressed in his trademark skinny jeans and trainers, his curly grey hair rampant, his shirt open and a small, drilled coin on an old bit of string around his neck – was in full flow that day. He was a great one for a lengthy exposition, but if he was at the wheel it detracted from the keen skill he had for pinpointing a police radar. Our first speeding ticket came not long after we left the main road.

'I grew up in Newnan, just south-west o'Atlanta, kind o' place there's two kinda folks: white folks an' black folks. Being a lawyer's like being a translator, 'cause that's what you do, really, act like a messenger between the prosecution and the defendant. Yeah, they sure do speak different languages, and I mean that literal . . .'

Millard began to wax lyrical on the job he loved. 'Lawyer's gotta be able to talk with judges and talk with normal folks. Too many don't talk to one or the other, then they can't help because they're lost in one of the worlds. Even a cheap office like ours at Team Defense has everything too *os-ten-ta-tious*.' The several syllables in the word were spat forward at the windscreen. Nobody could ever accuse Millard's torn trousers of looking ostentatious. 'I'd like to see us wear blue jeans in court . . . the suits we wear are just a mask, a costume, so we're play-acting fo' them other folks that's there, trying to live in the world o' the judge. Them suits don't represent who we really are, but if we don't wear them, the judge don't even begin to listen to us, 'cause we're not in his world.'

This road trip was, to me, meant to be research for my seminal book that would bring everyone to their senses about the death penalty. Listening to Millard, and seeing the men on death row who had no right to a lawyer unless they could afford one, belatedly brought me around to the recognition that I'd better get a law degree. It took me a while truly to identify the right lessons though. I wanted to be Millard, but I could not hope to emulate him: I could barely follow the construction of his Georgia grammar. He laughed loudly when I suggested I could learn from him – and told me I had to learn to be me if I wanted to do any good.

My problem with that was I was not sure who I was – half the South appeared to think I wasn't speaking the same language as them. The hardest word of all, for reasons that continue to elude me, was 'water': I would stand in front of the fast-food counter asking for a simple glass of water, slurring the term in as many variations as possible, adding random d-noises, even trying H-2-Oh, getting no closer to slaking my thirst.

'You don't ever accept defeat . . . that's what I put my heart on,' was Millard's ultimate mantra. 'Nothing can't be pulled out o' the fire, if you'll excuse my phrasing it like that. Means, though, that you can't ever *hate* people. Worst prosecutor or judge I run across, I can't *hate* him. No question about his motives, they're wrong – self-interest, greed for public acknowledgement, ignorance maybe – but he's just a china plate with cracks in it, like a criminal who does wrong. Y'know what, you can't want to help some folks an' then be punitive to others if their problem's the same. An' they're both plates that got cracked somewhere along the line, an' I think how maybe it could've happened to me. An' I think how it don't take nothing but glue to mend broken china.'

He got introspective. He'd been down to a Georgia execution. There is invariably the bride's side and the groom's side out by the pine trees, where the demonstrators are kept apart by the police – some praying for an eleventh-hour stay of execution, the others baying for blood. Millard had been walking between them to be with his client for those final minutes when he spotted someone in the crowd he knew, a guy he'd been friends with in high school. The man was behind the pro-death barrier, his face contorted like Edvard Munch's *The Scream*. Millard said he didn't hate the man; for a moment he saw who he might have become.

'Yeah, y'know what, I can see how I was cracked china too one time, wearing a suit and tie then too. I don't think I was so different that I was ever *for* the death penalty – I can't remember that – but there was times I just didn't think about it, and that's as bad. I wanted to be a great attorney, up there fencing with the best of them, and making lots of money, when I should've been paying more careful attention to others . . . what was happening in the larger view of things.'

Millard had thought about the idiosyncrasies of the people around him, and he was always working on a way to get them to do the right thing. 'It's real important for y'all to see that this ain't no different from the folks I'm defending, the men on death row – they're wrong too, sometimes, and they can be got right just the same. But it's real important too for y'all to see that there's more crime goes home with a coat and tie on each night than you'll ever find in the ghettos.'

I wondered for the first time whether a life like Millard's would suit Dad. Dad could certainly have argued well with judges, and his penchant for lateral thinking could have helped him deal with some of the madness of capital cases. I soon forgot about Dad in that respect, but I decided that at least it might fit my own temperament.

Back in Georgia, visiting Jack and the other men on death row, I kept on with my project for now, and each evening I would bash away at my prize possession, a blue Corona electric typewriter. Four months later, *Life on Death Row* was off to various publishers. I had just read John Kennedy Toole's *A Confederacy of Dunces* – his mother had eventually got it published eleven years after he took his own life in 1969. He won a posthumous Pulitzer. I harboured similar ambitions for my book, though I hoped to remain alive.

Unsurprisingly, the rejection slips trickled in. At least Jack Potts liked it, and my constant attention had kept him happy to stay alive for some months, allowing Millard to do his job for other people. That was my only contribution.

It was clear that I'd better go to law school. I chose Columbia solely because it was in New York, a city that I had heard of.

11

Law School and Insanity

That he's mad, 'tis true: 'tis true 'tis pity,
And pity 'tis 'tis true: a foolish figure.
William Shakespeare, *Hamlet* (Act II, Scene 2)

The day I arrived on campus at Columbia Law School, all the students were in suits. This was the world Millard had warned me against. I worried that I was meant to dress that way the whole time – after all, at Radley we had worn jackets, ties, gowns and even ridiculous mortar boards each day – and I only had one light grey suit that was already wearing thin. I was relieved to discover they were dressed up for their law firm interviews, angling for a high-paid job the next summer.

I went along to a corporate law recruitment evening just once, at my roommate Doug Beasley's insistence that it was a way to get free drinks and good hors d'oeuvres. We were high up above Central Park South, each gaggle of law students assigned to one of the staff. Doug and I were admiring the view in the dying sunlight when the young associate tasked with talking us into a life with Morgan Lewis suggested what a great place it would be to leap to one's death.

The sociopathy of the law students reminded me of the stereotype of the 'criminal'. If there was a question in class that depended on reading a particular legal decision, it was common to find that the case had been razored out of the relevant volume in the library by someone intent on being the only one to get the answer right. On the professional ethics exam, one of my classmates was commended for carefully explaining how each part of his proposed legal advice to his client was unethical. Within days of my arrival, I was co-editor of the newspaper, the *Law School News*, as nobody wanted the job – it was a distraction from gaining a corporate future. My co-editor wrote the kind of articles that interested most of the students, about job prospects for graduates. The previous year, 91 per cent had taken jobs in law firms or clerkships with judges, a few were disillusioned with the law altogether, and just 3 per cent (nine people out of three hundred) were doing 'public service', which included prosecuting people and working in Congress.

With my picayune power as co-editor, I was wont to rant. The legal education contemplated by Columbia gave me little that was of any use in my chosen field, and the effort to make us write 'efficiently' merely threatened to ruin whatever style we had. The bible of legal method was *Plain English for Lawyers*, taking most of the beauty out of writing while mandating pompous Latin phrases that would impress fee-paying clients.

In a petty rebellion, I wrote 'Plain Shakespeare for Lawyers', as I imagined law school would have taught the greatest poet in history to edit his work. 'Extancy's efficacy depends on the relative anguish of misfortune versus death. Suicide has completive attraction, but possible drawbacks.' The first half of Hamlet's entire soliloquy down to eighteen words, replacing the ninety-seven used by the Verbose Bard. I begged readers to consider the statistical significance of this methodology: a lengthy play cut to thirty minutes. With a takeout dinner eaten in the limousine, a corporate lawyer could be back at his desk in forty-five minutes.

I had only one goal, which was to return to Georgia as soon as I could, to help Millard with his mission. It was not as easy as I imagined. An education at Columbia could leave you $100,000 in debt – the equivalent of a 1984 mortgage without the house. No NGO, scraping by, was going to pay anything for a recent graduate who knew nothing to come and work for them. I had to figure out how to avoid all these loans, and then somehow come up with my own salary.

Meanwhile, one of the furious debates that I provoked in the *Law School News* involved the insanity defence. The majority of US states at the time still applied the M'Naghten Rule for insanity, which had been around since 1843 when Daniel M'Naghten planned to assassinate British prime minister Robert Peel but instead shot Peel's secretary, Edward Drummond. M'Naghten was a curious character. He grew up in Glasgow, and fell out with his father, a joiner. After a failed career as an actor, he set up his own joinery business and did remarkably well, although he was more interested in his own radical politics. The Tories were out to get him, he insisted, but his family and colleagues paid little attention to his conspiracy theories.

Thus far, he reminded me of Dad.

He sold his successful company and went to London, where he strode up behind Drummond and shot him in the back. Drummond's wounds were far from fatal, but the contemporary medical intervention involved bloodletting, and this contributed to his death a few days later. The murder trial was the sensation of the season and M'Naghten faced the noose.

When he appeared before the Bow Street magistrate, M'Naghten made a brief statement to the assembled media. 'The Tories in my native city have compelled me to do this. They follow, persecute me wherever I go, and have entirely destroyed my peace of mind,' he declared. 'It can be proved by evidence. That is all I have to say.' Again, this reminded me of Dad, who had insisted throughout his 'persecution' by Cambridge University that whatever position he took could be proven beyond any doubt if only he could find a fair tribunal.

Unlike my father, who had spurned the university's efforts to declare him not guilty by reason of his mental health, M'Naghten had a successful defence, both since he was relatively well-off and because there appears to have been a pre-existing move-ment among lawyers and doctors to update the arcane rules on legal insanity. At his trial, three respected doctors said his illness 'deprived him of all restraint over his actions', and the judge, Sir Nicholas Tindal, instructed the jury to acquit, with the proviso that proper care would be taken of him.

The case provoked outrage across the nation. Queen Vic-toria, who had been spooked by threats against her own royal personage, demanded that the House of Lords retry him – an idea that would have contravened the doctrine of double jeop-ardy. Instead, the Lords sent a series of questions to Chief Justice Tindal, who replied in terms that later became known as the M'Naghten Rule:

> The jurors ought to be told in all cases that every man is to be presumed to be sane, and to possess a sufficient degree of reason to be responsible for his crimes, until the contrary be proved to their satisfaction; and that to estab-lish a defence on the ground of insanity, it must be clearly proved that, at the time of the committing of the act, the party accused was labouring under such a defect of reason, from disease of the mind, as not to know the nature and quality of the act he was doing; or, if he did know it, that he did not know he was doing what was wrong.

This was all very well as judicial Victoriana, and it meant that M'Naghten spent the rest of his life in Bethlem and Broad-moor rather than ending it at the gallows. But it was a decision of its antiquarian day. Why, for example, should there be a pre-sumption of sanity with the burden of proof placed on a potentially insane individual, given that the prosecution bears the onus of proving the defendant guilty beyond a reasonable doubt? And why should someone be found guilty if they could not control his actions, regardless of whether they knew it was wrong (an 'irresistible impulse')? By the time I arrived in law school, M'Naghten had prevailed in the US for 140 years. There had been periodic efforts, generally led by the liberal elite judges in Washington, DC, to drag the law forward, with little ultimate impact.

In the 1950s, the DC Circuit Court of Appeal proposed the Durham Rule. In 1951, Monte Durham had been caught trespassing in a house. He had a long history of mental problems, starting when he was medically discharged from the navy in 1945, and running through a series of minor crimes for motor theft and bad cheques. He had periodically been sent to St Elizabeths Hospital, Washington's notorious forensic psychiatric institution built in 1855. In the late nineteenth century, when animals were brought over from Africa for the national zoo, they were sometimes housed there until they could be relocated. By the 1950s, as many as 8,000 people were warehoused in the wards. Once you were in, you might never get out – commitment there was said to be the only way to get a life sentence in DC. Alternatively, depending on the panel of doctors, you might be set free the next day.

Durham had been variously diagnosed with psychosis or psychopathic personality disorder, depending on the day and the doctor. His mother insisted that he suffered from hallucinations. Each time he was sectioned, the hospital – high on patients and low on public funds – would soon declare him fit and send him on his way, generally back to court, which is where he found himself in 1951.

'In view of the fact that he has been over there [St Elizabeths] a couple of times . . . I don't think I should take the responsibility of dropping these cases against him,' said the prosecutor to the trial judge. 'Then Saint Elizabeths would let him out on the street, and if that man committed a murder next week then it is my responsibility. So we decided to go to trial on one case, that is the case where we found him right in the house, and let him bring in the defense, if he wants to, of unsound mind at the time the crime was committed, and then

Your Honor will find him on that, and in your decision send him back to Saint Elizabeths Hospital, and then if they let him out on the street it is their responsibility.'

The judge was not going to roll the dice either, and sent Monte Durham to prison. By the time the case got to the court of appeals, he had already done three years.

The court appointed Abe Fortas to represent him. Fortas was a hero of the Bar who would later become a justice on the US Supreme Court. He persuaded the judges to fashion a new rule, where an 'accused is not criminally responsible if his unlawful act was the *product* of mental disease or some mental defect'. The aim of this was to bring the law in line with rapidly developing, yet hotly contested, notions of psychiatric medicine.

'The modern science of psychology,' Judge David Bazelon wrote, early in a career devoted to recasting the insanity defence, 'does not conceive that there is a separate little man in the top of one's head called reason whose function it is to guide another unruly little man called instinct, emotion, or impulse in the way he should go.' Every aspect of the accused's mind should be viewed together – though even he did not differentiate between the rich and the poor, those who had been fortunate enough to receive a good education and those who had not. Meanwhile, the Court came up with a broad and vague definition of 'mental illness': 'any abnormal condition of the mind which substantially affects mental or emotional processes and substantially affects behaviour controls'.

I'm not sure what that means. My father certainly harboured views that were 'abnormal' according to the majority – but I suspect I do too, and perhaps Boris Johnson and Donald Trump do as well. The court was dissatisfied for different reasons, and some years later, in 1972, it tinkered some more.

After drinking all afternoon, Archie Brawner got into a brawl with some inebriated neighbours, and came away with a broken jaw. Angry, he went home for his gun and returned, firing five times through the metal door of the apartment. By chance, two of the bullets hit Billy Ford, who died.

The doctors all agreed that Brawner suffered from a neurological 'abnormality' (epilepsy) and a 'personality disorder' (variously described as 'explosive' or 'convulsive'), which left him more likely to lose control, and which had been exacerbated by both alcohol and a blow to the face.

The problem with the Durham Rule, eight of the DC judges thought, was that it gave too much power to the experts. Everyone might agree that someone was psychotic, but then a battery of experts would battle over whether the illness had 'produced' the crime. Somehow, their new definition was meant to cure this. 'If, at the time of the criminal conduct, the defendant, as a result of mental disease or defect, either lacked substantial capacity to conform his conduct to the requirements of the law, or lacked substantial capacity to appreciate the wrongfulness of his conduct,' they wrote, he should be found not guilty by reason of insanity.

Judge Bazelon – who had written the Durham Rule – was the lone dissenter. 'This court's search for a new set of words to define the elusive concept of responsibility has a distinctly archaic quality,' he wrote. 'What should by now be clear is that the problems of the responsibility defense cannot be resolved by adopting any new formulation of words. The practical operation of the defense is primarily controlled by other factors, including the quality of counsel, the attitude of the trial judge, the ability of the expert witnesses, and the adequacy of the pretrial mental examination.'

All the judges (even Bazelon) ignored the tableau on which Archie Brawner's life was drawn, and focused on the minutes before the shooting as if they were a ring-fenced scene on television, unrelated to the myriad episodes of his life that had gone before.

Meanwhile the case saw an interesting tiff between America's psychiatrists and psychologists, who intervened to give the court the benefit of their perspective. The American Psychiatric Association wanted to abolish the insanity defence altogether, send everyone to prison and then treat them. There might be more merit to this position if we only sent people to prison who were genuinely dangerous to our society, and treated them properly while seeking a cure. Additionally, the psychiatrists vehemently believed that psychologists should not be permitted to testify. 'Psychologists study philosophy, not medicine,' they declared. 'They have PhD degrees – i.e., doctors of philosophy.' They insisted that the entire debate should be left to *real* doctors.

Meanwhile, the American Psychological Association did take a much more philosophical line. They argued that the court should not distinguish between 'physiological, emotional, social or cultural' sources for any impairment in Brawner's ability to control himself: 'If a defendant is unable to control his conduct, there is no basis in science or morality to distinguish between physiological or medical causes for the condition and social or emotional causes.'

This made sense to the psychologists – and it makes sense to me – but it exposes the gulf between human behaviour and the law. The entire legal system is premised on a notion that there are various reasons to punish someone. In law school these were clearly defined for us. First, there is retribution – the idea that we should punish people for the simple reason that they *should* be punished. This is a purely philosophical concept, with nothing to do with medicine or objectivity. It runs contrary to my entirely subjective view: I have never punished my son for anything, since it seems like a failing in the way I have brought him up if I did not impart a moral compass to him in a compassionate way.

Second, there is deterrence. This justified public hangings, where the spectacle of a criminal on the end of a rope was meant to deter others from the same act. In his study *The*

Deterrence Hypothesis and Picking Pockets at the Pickpocket's Hanging, David Anderson begins with the old trope of how pickpockets worked the crowd while one of their colleagues was being hanged. Anderson suggested that 89 per cent of violent criminals do not stop to think about the consequences of their actions – should they even be sober enough at the time to do so. Deterrence is, in my experience, generally a myth: the possibility of being punished never occurs to most of my clients. Neither do you and I abstain from murder because we are afraid of the forthcoming trial – we decide not to kill someone because we have been imbued with the idea that it is not a good thing to do.

Closely related, there is the idea of 'specific deterrence' – where we are supposedly deterring the individual from doing this again. This may have fitted with an era when children were taught at the end of a cane – 'spare the rod, spoil the child'. Yet today we tend to think in terms of teaching the child, rather than beating them: 'there's no such thing as a bad dog, only a bad dog owner' is a more modern motto.

Then there is the most flawed notion of all – that the victim somehow needs the perpetrator to be punished for the victim's mental well-being. This is a very sorry concept, where we tell people they will feel better if they insist on revenge.

As a society, we tend to accept the concept of punishment without bothering with the theoretical underpinnings. To me, this is one of the mad notions that is firmly embraced by 95 per cent of our social order. In law school, it was even worse: we were told to accept and then squeeze it into as many of the philosophical boxes as we could, rather than standing back for a moment and wondering whether the whole process made sense. When I look over my lifetime, the extent to which we have abandoned the harsh punishment of children in favour of educational encouragement is one of the extraordinary advances of modern society. I was waterboarded in school; someone who slaps a child in a supermarket today is likely to be brought up on charges. Whether we are going to extend our generosity of spirit to children once they are grown is another matter, but it is worth considering.

The psychologists did indeed want a philosophical debate, and they were right to do so. Archie Brawner got into a fight when he was drunk. His drinking was linked to an alcohol addiction, and it interacted with his neurological idiosyncrasy. By definition, this was a large part of his failure to control himself. American law simply ignores this, telling us that he was 'voluntarily' intoxicated. Therefore it is deemed that he should have foreseen all the possible consequences of drinking. While the pain from his recently broken jaw was also a precipitating factor, the law deems that equally irrelevant. The law simply ignores human reality.

'The magic of medical categories and their technical jargon retains its considerable power to obscure both thought, and the biographical facts of the defendant's case,' wrote the psychologists. If Brawner did not come from a poor family, live in a poor neighbourhood and have little or no family support, the chances of him getting into such violent encounters would fall precipitously. For all my own idiosyncrasies, I would almost certainly not have shot someone under similar circumstances in England, because I had been conditioned at boarding school to have a very high threshold before losing my temper – and I would anyway not have been living in a country where everyone has access to a gun.

'The concept of normality has become the criterion for mental health. But since the middle class is most often the source of what is considered "normal", we are in peril of utilising "mental health" to perpetuate middle-class values,' the psychologists concluded.

The judges ignored everything the psychologists had to say. The bickering between the judges over the semantic definition of 'insanity' was a theoretical debate, without any link to the real world. What did it mean to have what was called a 'mental defect'? If you read the *Diagnostic and Statistical Manual of Mental Disorders*, you will find me (and perhaps yourself) in at least twenty diagnostic categories, from drinking more than seven measures of alcohol a week on upwards.

When Dad told me to go live by myself when I was seven years old, did he 'appreciate the wrongfulness of his conduct'? Dad would have pointed to the British elite, who were sending their children away to boarding school at that age. At least one president of the United States probably thought there was nothing wrong – that it is flattering to a woman – if he 'grabs her by the pussy'. In other words, the insanity defence encompasses many things. It also captures nothing, since virtually nobody prevails in a real courtroom because jurors are so loath to 'excuse' someone from punishment by finding them insane.

Perhaps we should not be thinking about vague definitions of sanity. While the psychologists made a good deal more sense, perhaps the psychiatrists were half right: we should focus rather on whether someone is dangerous and 'curable'. If we did away with the idea that we should punish someone for punishment's sake, and instead kept our eyes firmly on whether they are a threat to society, the judicial process would achieve a sensible purpose. We might even begin to treat people we don't know in the same way we would treat those we love.

This debate prompted my next adolescent sally into saving the world from itself. Bob Goldstein was a medical doctor in our class, a mature student who was getting a doctoral degree in law so he could do medical malpractice cases, which were immensely lucrative at the time. He had a splendid apartment down Broadway where one evening he assembled people for a debate about the 'Psychopathic Murderer'. The majority were heavily inclined towards the idea of 'evil', comfortable to join the psychiatrists in getting rid of the insanity defence altogether. I was their vociferous opponent, regarded with a mixture of fondness and condescension by my elders.

Inevitably I inflicted my views on the entire student body in the *Law School News*, and then expanded it into a stolid article in the *Human Rights Law Review*. Did people not understand that Cicero had discussed the insanity defence in *Tusculanae Disputationes* in 45 BCE? Cnut and Æthelred the Unready had recognised the defence. The annals of Henry VII contained an entire capital trial held in 1506 described in four pithy sentences, which would surely have made the authors of our legal-method textbook proud: '*Un home fuit arreine de murder d'un enfant. Et trouve fuit q al teps del murd le felon fuit de non saine memoire. Par q~ ag fuit, q~ il ira quite. Quod nota bene.*' ('A man was arraigned for the murder of a child. It was found that at the time of the murder the felon was not sane. For which reason he was acquitted. Note well.') We'd had the defence forever, I said, and it would be barbaric to be rid of it.

Recently, I looked up the history of my article to evaluate the impact my research had had upon the world: I discovered that in thirty-five years my words of wisdom had not been cited by anyone at all – not even, most surprisingly, by myself.

Cristiana Ferraro, an *elegantissima* Italian, had been trying to translate her relationship with her father, Francesco, who had emigrated to New York, into her right to remain in the US. Her application was mired in the habitual chaos of the Immigration and Naturalization Service (INS), and she was in danger of being thrown out of the country. Confused, she had come to our free Columbia clinic close to the end of my rather tedious legal degree. We soon navigated the path between the various bureaucrats and got her green card in hand.

I was thrilled to have Cristiana as a 'client', though the clinic later used our case as an ethics scenario to discuss when student lawyers could cross professional boundaries with someone they were meant to be helping. At the time, the morality of it never occurred to me. Cristiana and I were the same age, legal 'aliens' from Europe caught up in the alien world of New York. She was – is – the sophisticated daughter of a stockbroker father (Francesco had been a conservative in Italy, then remarried in America, where he found himself a liberal) and an accountant mother, Renata (still back in Milan). In classic Italian style, Renata was a bourgeois member of the Stalinist Party: I later noticed Cristiana's photograph on the mantelpiece with another of her well-coiffed sister Francesca, on either side of a framed portrait of Uncle Joe.

I was intrigued by Cristiana's glamour. I loved my scarlet jacket; she politely shuddered. She favoured the arcades near Milan's Duomo – all name labels, all far beyond either my budget or my aspirations. She wore her dark hair in a 1920s bob, curving around a circular face, and strode the streets of New York with her back straight and her Milanese shoes slightly splayed.

'Clive and I met in New York towards the end of May 1984,' she later described it to a journalist, in her light Italian accent. 'We met in very interesting circumstances. He was helping people with immigration problems, and I happened to be one of them. We met at Federal Plaza. We had to wait a long time at the INS office and Clive and I talked and laughed. He made jokes about the immigration laws and the immigration officers. I thought lawyers were boring, serious people. It was a time I enjoyed immensely because the unpleasant atmosphere of that office was turned into a rather romantic setting. A movie in the old-fashioned style, a bit like *Casablanca*.

'I was fascinated by Clive's ease at dealing with the immigration people; he did all the talking. I can understand what some of Clive's clients on death row felt, it was a feeling of hope,' she went on, somewhat overstating my role. Actually, the immigration officer was studying law at night school. He was rather overawed that I was at a posh place like Columbia, and when I offered up a few ideas for his homework we spent more time on that than on Cristiana's case, which was then in the bag.

'The next thing I know is that after we were through and

out of the building with a strong feeling of lightness,' Cristiana continued, the way she used to speak, in occasional phrases that I found attractively odd. 'We went walking in Central Park in the rain, eating an ice cream which I remember Clive, in a moment of nervousness, dropped on his trousers, resulting in him flushing and calling himself a fool. In this rainy day it was bright and hilarious. It was the beginning of something good for me and I invited Clive to lunch at my parents' place the day after. I still remember how I came home talking to my father and my stepmother Rita about how I never had before such a wonderful time at the immigration office.'

It was true. I was nervous. Though I was twenty-four, I had never been in a meaningful relationship. I had spent my entire life from eight to eighteen in bizarre unisex boarding schools with their inattention to the real world. Even after three years as an undergraduate and another three in law school, Cristiana was the first person I had met with whom I felt aligned, perhaps because of our classic European sense of scepticism at many things American. Her case was the last I worked on before graduating, and when I headed off to New Orleans to take the Louisiana Bar exam she tagged along.

I had helped to set up a loan forgiveness programme – much more generous in 1984 than Britain proposes today, forgiving everything after seven years in the public service – and I had extracted a grant from Columbia's Public Interest Law Foundation, made up of tithes paid by the graduates who had gone to corporate law firms. My plan was to survive for the whole year on their $3,500, and so I had offered my services to Team Defense. To my great sorrow, Millard told me that he was teetering so close to bankruptcy that they could not even promise to be there.

I turned to Steve Bright, who headed the Southern Prisoners Defense Committee (SPDC), another tiny charity in Atlanta. Steve took me on faith. He planned ahead, thinking that we ought to open a Louisiana office, since that was where the Fifth

Circuit Court of Appeals was located – 'the buckle of the Death Belt' covering Mississippi, Louisiana and Texas. Hence Cristiana and I took the Trailways bus from New York to a Mennonite home on St Andrew Street, New Orleans. The Mennonites were, like the Quakers, friends of the anti-death-penalty movement, and we paid $100 a month for a small room with a mattress on the floor, along with a stray calico kitten who had wandered by. We named her Tchoupitoulas Ferraro after our favourite New Orleans street and Cristiana's surname, which is the equivalent of 'Smith' in Italian, a language in which all words sound more attractive. (After all, Giuseppe Verdi translates as Joe Green.)

'We are having a great time,' I wrote to my mother, 'notwithstanding the increasingly dark cloud of the Bar exam looming above me . . .' I ignored my studies while we enjoyed ourselves on our meagre budget, alternating long walks by the Mississippi with inexpensive ventures into the French Quarter oyster bars. I was not really motivated to prepare, as I was not sure I would be allowed to sit the exam. The Louisiana Bar Association said that as an 'alien' I could not take it, so I was forced to sue them, alleging a violation of the right to equal protection of the law, with the $75 filing fee almost a month's food budget. When my law school insurance ran out, I decided not to pay even for minimal health coverage, which would have cost $100 a month. I immediately got ill and had to pay $60 for medication. Meanwhile the Mennonites left for good, leaving us to pay for the whole house. Peter, a born-again Christian and a firm adherent to the principle that Jesus would provide, showed up at the door. His endless sermons were irritating, and Jesus had apparently designated us as proxy so Peter consumed our limited stocks of food and drink.

The afternoon before Independence Day, I learned that I had won my case against the Bar Association. While that was my first glorious courtroom victory, it did mean I had no excuse to avoid knuckling down for the last two weeks before the test. I had to choose a pseudonym as well, as Louisiana's long history of corruption included the invigilators adding some points for people they knew. I agonised with Cristiana: I leaned towards Karl Marx, but she thought that would be an automatic fail. I settled on John Stuart Mill, since someone told me he had the highest IQ of anyone who ever lived, and I needed the help. Soon after the exam, we rode the bus to Atlanta, where I met Steve Bright for the first time and started work with the SPDC. Within a week I already had half a dozen capital cases.

The evening before Cristiana left to head back to the Big Apple, I got my Bar results. Somehow I had passed all ten subjects, which did not speak well of the quality of law in Louisiana. We went for a drink in the revolving restaurant at the top of the Peachtree Plaza Hotel. In the hour it took us to drink one overpriced cocktail, we got to see all 360 degrees of the city.

'A few centuries from now,' Alain de Botton writes in *The Course of Love*, 'the level of self-knowledge that our own age judges necessary to get married might be thought puzzling, if not outright barbaric. By then, a standard, wholly non-judgemental line of enquiry (appropriate even on a first date), to which everyone would be expected to have a tolerant, good-natured and non-defensive answer, would simply be: "So in what ways are you mad?"'

My mother had no idea whom she was marrying when Dad proposed to her outside the old Fulbourn Asylum. Likewise, Cristiana deserved to be told, in forthright terms, that if she married me, it would be bigamous, as I was already married to my job. It should have been explained to her that I had been sent away to boarding school, and had therefore had all emotions crammed into a very small guarded compartment deep within my psyche. There were a few things I might have been warned about too. I will never regret our marriage, but we had no concept of our differences.

12

The Gassing of Edward Earl Johnson

O what made fatuous sunbeams toil
To break Earth's sleep at all?

Wilfred Owen, 'Futility'

For the first year of our relationship, I tried to get to New York when I could. My mother sent me Trailways bus vouchers that allowed twenty-four hours of travel in any direction around America for just $10. New York was just in range, and I went there once a month, leaving on a Thursday evening with a briefcase full of someone's trial transcript, and arriving at Port Authority twenty-one hours later, before returning over Sunday night.

After a year Cristiana moved to Atlanta, and went to Emory University to try to locate her passion. We decided to get married, and we set the date for 14 February 1986. That was my idea. What I did not know at the time is that, statistically, people who get married on Valentine's Day are more likely to get divorced.

Dad was fairly high around this time. The first indicator was that he announced that he had decided to work for no money forever. The insulting letters about his useless kids were another sign. It took about a month for him to respond to my letter announcing our engagement.

'I am certain that marriage as an institution is outdated and on balance it destroys rather than creates love, but it is probably with us for the rest of the century,' he replied. 'And with Cristiana's Italian and Roman Catholic background probably that makes marriage the best solution. In any case, you have my blessing and wholehearted support.' With this he was through with the issue of marriage, and it was time to get on to other matters. 'What would seem of greater concern is what you are going to do with your life since you are clearly wasting it now.'

The gulf between my world and Cristiana's became clear with the execution date that came down a year later in the case of Edward Earl Johnson. I had been spending a lot of time in Mississippi and I had encountered him in passing on my visits to the prison. I knew he was slightly younger even than me, a black kid who had been sentenced to die when he was eighteen for supposedly killing a white town marshal. The word on the row was that he did not do it. When Edward got a date, I called his lawyer Ken Rose in Jackson to offer help. Edward had somehow slipped through the first round of appeals: the federal courts had rejected Ken's arguments for a new trial and we would be in what is called a 'successor' posture, with Edward now having to show not only that he'd had an unfair trial, but that he had some excuse for failing to raise this the first time around. Rob McDuff, a brilliant lawyer and a good friend, also piled in.

We had only three weeks to the execution date, but that was not rare. For my part, there was an abundance of youthful arrogance: I had yet to lose a client to execution in the all of three years since I left law school, and I saw no reason to start with Edward. Paul Hamann, a director with the BBC, had contacted me about a death penalty film he was making called *Fourteen Days in May*, and he said he had access to Parchman Penitentiary to follow the two weeks running up to the execution on the twentieth of the month. I said it would be a welcome distraction for Edward, but I was sure we would ruin the ending of the film by getting a stay of execution.

Cristiana was not happy. She was afraid to stay home alone, she said, but I could not really see that she had much to worry about. I had boasted to my mother about the iron bars I had found in a wreck yard that now sealed all the downstairs windows, along with the big red alarm bell high on the front wall of the two-storey house.

I don't remember a great deal about those three weeks in 1987. I know I spent long hours reading the transcript and writing lengthy pleadings. I thought legal issues were more important than factual investigation – the hardest element of my failure, over the years, has been the knowledge that I got that all wrong.

I had been in Mississippi for ten days, and was in Ken's office late on a Friday night, when I got an urgent call from Cristiana in Atlanta. She was very upset. She had been out, and come back to our house on Glenwood Avenue to find the front door smashed off its hinges. She was going to a friend's house for the night.

It was a rather desperate moment in Edward's case, but I promised to set out for home early in the morning.

I was on the road by 5.30 a.m., rather a danger to myself and others as I drove the 128 miles up to Parchman – I had to check in with Edward to tell him that I had an emergency. Don Cabana was a very decent prison warden, and he got me a cup of dreadful coffee at the same time as authorising an unscheduled client visit at 8 a.m. I drove five hundred yards into the prison, turned left on the dirt track to Unit 27, and put my car keys in the plastic bucket lowered by the guard in the tower. Edward was nonchalant about his lawyer doing house repairs for a fifth of the time left before his scheduled execution. I then drove the 403 miles that I knew so well back to Atlanta and arrived in the early afternoon to find Cristiana inside and the front door splintered all down the jamb. We went immediately to a Home Depot store so we could select the strongest oak door, along with a metal grille, that would better defend the entrance.

As I worked late into the night putting the doorway back

together, she sat on the arm of the nearby chair with a glass of red wine and we talked.

'Any idea what has gone missing?' I asked her at one point. She had not mentioned anything, and I was not sure she had faced up to it.

It turned out that she had. 'Yes,' she said. 'Do you promise you won't be mad at me?'

'Of course,' I said. 'Why on earth would I?'

'Well,' she began tentatively, 'they took the television, and two pieces of jewellery . . . You know my red brooch? . . . And my wedding ring.' She looked a little nervous. I did not understand. 'You see, I had taken it off to go out for the evening with my friends.'

I eventually understood. It was hardly a big deal. I knew what she meant. Men tend to have a stupid idea that married women are out of bounds for dancing and even talking. I was not annoyed at her for doing it, I just thought she was very unlucky. What were the odds of them stealing just that, quite safely hidden near our bed upstairs, on the one night she had taken it off? My only sorrow was that it had belonged to my favoured grandmother, Vera, and been on her finger for the half-century that she had been married – and now some arsehole was going to pawn it for $20. I'd have happily given them ten times that amount, no questions asked, to have it back.

Losing in the federal district court in Jackson, Mississippi, was a hard blow. It was noon on Tuesday, 19 May 1987, and Edward still had at least twelve hours of life, until one minute past midnight. Late the previous evening, we had held a hearing. It had gone well, and although they would not let Edward come to play a part in his fate, I had been able to give him hope afterwards in a telephone call. The next morning, the judge called us into his chambers and denied Edward's petition. Later, when I read his judgement carefully, the intellectual dishonesty of it all made my blood boil. It came down to the deranged idea that the legal system would be diminished if Edward was allowed to keep on appealing.

I took the notice of appeal downstairs in the same building myself, to deliver it to Judge Charles Clark of the Fifth Circuit Court of Appeals. Edward had pulled one of the most conservative three-judge panels from the dozen members of the circuit. There was little hope that we would find relief there – but all hope, and much faith in the legal system, vanished when I entered his chambers. His secretary recognised me as Edward's attorney and stood, obviously nervous, in front of the printer, which only served to draw my attention there. When she turned away, I could see that Judge Clark had already written the opinion denying relief and was printing it out before we had even lost in the district court. It was only noon and yet, to preserve the appearance of justice, the secretary told me that the court would not decide until about 6 p.m. – and no, they would not permit me to argue on Edward's behalf.

The Supreme Court and the governor were the only chances left.

Rob McDuff had flown to Washington early that morning, to be ready to file our appeal to the Supreme Court. It was a strange waste of money that we did not have: the court rules had not yet caught up with the existence of the fax machine. Soon after I left the district court, I set off on that 128-mile drive up to the prison again, to be with Edward. I found him in a small room to the left of the entrance to death row, with all his family. After a while, with time dragging, I looked for a way to distract everyone. I asked him whether he would like a game of chess. The guards let me go and get his board from his cell, and we set up the pieces. As if we were just playing to pass the time one quiet evening, Edward made me look like a beginner.

Then he had to hug his family goodbye – his mother, his wizened and wonderful old granny, all his sisters. I was allowed to stay, along with his spiritual adviser, Sandy, and we were taken to Edward's cell, past thirteen other men condemned to die in that same gas chamber, which was just beyond the door at the end. All the men lined along the row were Edward's friends, and several were my clients. Sam Johnson, another black man there for supposedly killing a white police officer, smiled with encouragement as we passed, but I could see the sadness lining his dark eyes. It was not looking good.

We waited outside Edward's cell for the guard to open it with the electric control. Then Edward, Sandy and I were locked inside his little world with just a rose Sandy had brought for him, letters from well-wishers, and a battered TV on the metal shelf at the end of the bed – a link to the world outside, so far away. Edward flipped the knob. The announcer was intoning that 'inmate Edward Earl Johnson' had lost in the district court, and I felt my customary irritation that everyone else should be called 'Mr' – a peculiar lack of respect.

A guard told me there was a telephone call. Edward looked up at me as I left the cell. I walked briskly out to the tiny, sweaty room near the front gate. When I picked up the receiver, at first there was no response. Finally, I could hear Rob's voice fading in from the background. Seven to two against, he said, only Brennan and Marshall dissenting, as they did in every death penalty case. Justice Brennan had written a four-page dissent on one issue we had raised. I knew they had been our last real hope. Still, even if I had never been in this position before, I knew that my main job now was to keep on giving Edward hope, to help him through the final hour and a half.

I walked slowly back to the cell, through the clashing metal of the sliding prison gates. It was strange, surreal. I could feel my pink cotton shirt sticking to my back, the BBC camera following me somewhere further behind, off in another universe.

'So, it's up to the governor,' I told Edward when I got back to the cell. Governor Allain was Catholic, and we had the Pope himself intervening, I said. That much was true: a simple call to the Papal Legate in Washington, and within a couple of days the Pope had sent a message calling for mercy. I went through the reasons why the governor ought to grant clemency – no flattery, simple truth. (Not the whole truth: since the death penalty had become so politicised in the late 1970s, the use of clemency had dropped from almost one in three capital cases to something close to negligible.) I told him of all the good people who had intervened on his behalf. Edward squeezed my hand. Gradually we drifted back to talking about the letters he had received. Each of his friends had sent him a stamp, so that he would be able to reply to them the next day.

When the guard came to say that there was another call for me, I clapped Edward's shoulder and walked back up the block. When you think you are about to get a dreadful exam result . . . when you are waiting for a call from hospital . . . any attempt to explain the sensation trivialises it. Ken Rose came on the phone from Jackson. He said we had lost in the Supreme Court. Momentarily, a surge of relief came over me – I already knew that.

Then: 'The governor denied.' So expected, yet so harsh. How to move? How to go and tell Edward that it had been decreed that he should die? The hardest moment in my life.

What a thought! Edward was to die, and I was thinking of how difficult it was for me to tell him. Ridiculous. I walked back, at first with slow, aching steps. But then I remembered the other men on the block, and I knew I could not bow my head. Surrender by me would be surrender for them. I had been taught that appearances mattered. For many, I was meant to be their main source of hope as well. I therefore quickened as I entered the cell block, walked to his door, and sat on the bed next to him.

'He turned us down.' Edward seemed totally unmoved. Sandy suggested that we should pray. She said things which perhaps some can believe, and from which perhaps Edward drew strength. I found it small comfort to be told that some god had a purpose for this senseless barbarism.

Soon they moved us all to the 'preparation cell', and we sat on another hard mattress, facing a simple wooden crucifix. The BBC director Paul Hamann pretended to be interested in who made the cross. Another inmate, said Warden Cabana. Edward still talked about hope; Sandy read some more verses from the Bible concerning how God is with us in heaven as well as on earth.

Cabana, who I suspect abhorred the death process as much as anyone, tried to be human. 'Edward, I have to tell you that I have a tremendous amount of respect for you,' he said. 'And you'll remember what you promised me? You'll put in a good word for me with the man upstairs?'

I could see his transparent good intentions, but it seemed so alien. He left for a few moments, which seemed interminable. When he returned, he presented the strangest monologue of all.

'Edward, when we take you inside they're going to have to attach some little round . . . I forget what they call them . . . some . . . do–hickeys that they have . . . go to the electrocardiograph machine and they may need to remove a little hair. That'll happen at about a quarter till. We've got about twenty minutes until the medics come in and about seventeen minutes until we remove you from the room, OK? OK I just want you to know what they're doing.'

Edward was sitting there calmly, nodding as Cabana spoke, and everyone else was just listening as if it were really quite normal to talk about how the monitor would be hooked up to make sure he had been gassed to death. Against reality, even I began to expect someone to call an end to it and tell Edward he could come home with me.

Edward turned to Cabana. 'Mr Cabana, I just want to thank you for everything you've done for me.'

I was close to weeping at that moment, but I could not let myself go.

We sat together again for a while, and I held an arm tightly around Edward's shoulders, while Sandy gripped his hand.

Edward looked straight ahead. 'I suppose everyone wonders what a man thinks when he is about die,' he said quietly. 'Well, it ain't over till it's over.'

Paul Hamann said he felt the TV crew should leave. He emerged from behind the camera that he had been directing for two weeks. He hugged Edward. I suppose the camera went off, though nobody called 'cut'. Then the 'medical technicians' came in, and told Edward to lift up his shirt. I'm glad Edward did not look at me at that moment. How could those sworn to save lives assist in this gruesome ritual? They took heavy grey binding tape which one might use to secure a parcel and wrapped it twice tightly around Edward's chest. He even helped, politely holding it for them, as one of those faceless men then shaved a little hair next to each of Edward's shoulders and attached the ECG contacts.

I was grateful that Sandy had the forethought to tell Edward to put his blue shirt back on, restoring his dignity after this horrible scene. He just smiled, saying they had done it rather tightly, and maybe they wanted to suffocate him already?

Almost immediately, Cabana came back in. 'It's time, son.'

Edward kissed Sandy goodbye on her cheek. He turned to me. I said, no, I would come with him. So we put an arm around each other's shoulders and walked in there. I didn't really have anyone's permission, but I didn't think Cabana would stop me.

In a dreadful way, I was glad to be there with him. There seemed to be a dozen grey-faced guards in the small area that surrounded the gas chamber. Neither I nor, I am sure, Edward had ever before seen the awful thing. I hoped I would never see it again. No description can capture the evil of the diver's death bell with four windows for the spectators.

We hugged each other. He whispered in my ear. I did not hear, and asked him to repeat it.

'Do you know something that I don't know?' He looked up at me dubiously.

For a moment I did not understand. Then it hit me – somehow, he thought I still knew something that would put a stop to all this. The TV cameras, the surreality, he thought it was all a movie . . . that they had not let him in on it, to make it seem real.

I mumbled something innocuous about him knowing more than I ever would. I hugged him again and stood there as they strapped him into that disgusting chair. I smiled and gave him a thumbs up. He smiled back at me. Then the guards told me I had to leave. The door led to the outside . . . to the bright halogen lights, and then the humidity. I felt an overwhelming urge not to follow the procedure that was making it so damned easy.

I walked over to where Sandy was standing – and she burst into tears, letting emotions from the hours of encouragement flood out. As we leaned against a van, its engine still hot from bringing some person who apparently wanted to be here, she sobbed that she could not go into the witness room. I told her that of course she should not – what purpose would it serve? I knew that I had to: once before, an execution had been stopped because they botched it, and the lawyer was there. Who knew what might happen? So I went.

I was the only person there for Edward. I was ushered to a chair near the red-and-black telephone, high at the back where I was behind everyone else. The air conditioner was on, a large black curtain covered the window into the chamber. I took off my glasses, and held my head with my hands, unable to believe that I was really witnessing Edward's execution.

There were five media people there. Three guards from the prison. The attorney for the prison whom I had met at a party a year before. And others I did not know. Nobody cared to look in my direction. If they did catch my eye, they turned away – ashamed, I liked to believe. Although the only ones who looked truly uncomfortable were the guards, who at least knew Edward. One media person did acknowledge my presence. He wanted an interview. I ignored him. Then the curtain was pulled open, and his interest was in the colour of Edward's shoes, the cloth of his trousers . . .

I was drawn between a desperate need to look at Edward and a terrible desire not to, so as not to rob him of his dignity at this most undignified moment – his back was towards us so he would not know. In the end, when he spoke, I had to raise my head.

'I guess they won't call,' he said in a clear voice. 'I guess they won't call.' Only now, only now, did the reality of this horrid nightmare come to him, and I could not help him.

I never looked again. I stared at the second hand on my watch and dissociated. But I could not understand what was going on – they just kept him sitting there for eight minutes, doing nothing.

'Please,' said Edward in the end, 'let's get it over with.' But the timetable apparently could not be changed. The telephone rang. As a fleeting hope crossed my mind, a guard said that was the signal for it to begin. I wondered later if the sound registered with Edward, and if for a second he hoped that this was the call that would save him. The next minutes were to be those upon which the media would dwell, describing the sound of Edward gasping for breath. I was far away. My portcullis had rattled down.

'The prisoner is officially dead.' As we left the room, there was an eager discussion among the witnesses. They had never seen anything like it. The same journalist tapped me on the shoulder, wanting my reaction. I ignored him.

My car was just outside the death unit. I had to drive over to the prison chapel where the family were assembled. They had to have known, but I was the one who confirmed it. Tears flowed, there were screams. I had no idea what I was meant to say.

Then I had one final duty: the press conference up near the prison gates. I could not leave him unrepresented. I leaned on the wall to one side while Warden Cabana took the podium.

147

'Ladies and gentlemen, at 12.06 a.m. on Wednesday, May 20th, Edward Earl Johnson was executed in the gas chamber here at the Mississippi State Penitentiary, in accordance with the sentence of the Circuit Court of Leake County,' Cabana started fluently. He had a prepared script, but it was only one sentence long. 'I'll be glad to take any questions you may have.'

The journalists were squatting all around on the cheap government carpet, underneath the beam of the television cameras, hands up like kindergarten children.

'Did he have any last statements?' shouted one.

'Yes, he did,' Cabana began, long breaks coming every two or three words now, as he struggled with emotion. 'He indicated . . . his innocence. And that he regretted the situation . . . But that he bore no ill will toward anyone. And he was thankful that . . . the process was coming to a close for himself and his family. And . . . er . . .' – he searched for a closing line – '. . . he stated . . . that he was *not guilty*.'

'How long was there between the time the crystals hit the tray and the time the monitor showed cardiac arrest?' said one waving hand, in a thick, mid-Mississippi accent.

'Between the time the crystals . . .' Cabana said, the gaps even longer now, '. . . between the time the gas struck his face . . . and the time cardiac arrest was pronounced was . . . approximately twelve minutes . . . He was unconscious within a minute.' That was nonsense. They had no idea when he was unconscious.

'Let's hear from the lawyer,' cried the same penetrating Southern voice. 'He knew him.'

I have no idea how I got to the microphone, but I did. I had nothing prepared, so I just said what came to me.

'I just came from talking to the family,' I began, since that is what had happened. Having dissociated from the world, I had made no effort to come back yet. 'I ask you . . . what was I meant to say? Why did it happen? I stayed with Edward . . .' I paused. I owed it to him to say this differently, to say it *right*. 'I had the *privilege* to stay with Edward . . . for the last hours of his life, and he was a lot more calm than I was. And all I can say is, when the family asked me why, all I could say was . . . it's a sick world . . . it's a sick world. Thank you.'

I even thanked them. And then I left. I went out to my car and I started driving back to Jackson. Other than it being where I had come from earlier in the day, I'm not sure why I was going there. I suppose it was closer than Atlanta. I hadn't slept more than three or four hours a night in three weeks. I hadn't slept at all for a couple of days. I was lethal. I came close to running off the road a few times. I had little idea what I was doing. Somehow I got to Ken's house in Jackson. Somehow, after sleeping a few hours, I got into the car and headed home to Atlanta.

13

Love, Violence and Divorce

I never forget. I never forgive. I can wait. I find it easy to harbor a grudge.

Tom Wolfe

When I got home, there was a letter from the grave. I had told Edward about Cristiana's fear of being alone. The mailman had just delivered a card to her from Edward, with a cartoon he had drawn of Walt Disney's Goofy hitching to 'Atlanta or Bust'. There was a poem penned inside: 'Though I'm away a thousand miles, / and leave loved ones behind, / the most important one I know / is always on my mind.' From a letter I had sent him, Edward had then traced my own signature – *Clive*. He had thought to do this when he was preparing for death.

What I had just witnessed was a choreographed act of sheer lunacy, where all the might that Mississippi could assemble had focused on taking a nice young black kid and murdering him. What made it more difficult was that many supposedly rational and seemingly decent people had conspired to carry it out. I had wrestled with myself, alone, for more than four hundred miles back from Jackson. A part of me wanted to hate; but a larger part wanted them all committed to Whitfield State Hospital for the mentally unwell.

I did not try to talk to Cristiana, or anyone else, about Edward. They had not been there. Most tellingly, I immediately tried to repress the memory. Two weeks later I was back in Mississippi, working on Nevin Kerr Whetstone, who was headed to trial, represented by my mate Jimmy Doug Shelton.

Jimmy had been to school with Elvis in Tupelo, and his tatty office had plywood scenes of his old classmate all over the walls, obscured by the piled boxes of legal records. We worked the case out pretty quickly for a sentence of life with parole, which went into the win column. Recently, I discovered that Nevin is still in prison over thirty years later, which makes it a questionable victory.

Because Jimmy had a finger in everything in north-east Mississippi, he kindly helped me find a new, rather garish gold ring for Cristiana at way below the market price, as I had saved him a fair amount of work.

Dad was in Spain at this time, sending successive missives about the definition of love. Languid in the bath, he was through with two marriages now. He wanted to understand what love was, and he was thinking himself to a logical answer. Finally, he had come up with the definition. 'Love,' he opined, 'is the yearning to feel the happiness and fulfilment of the loved one.'

When I first read it, this made sense enough to me. It was a long time before I realised that Dad's immersion in the idea of love was rather similar to the judges in the District of Columbia, with their effort to identify the standard of 'insanity': these were words. They were intellectual, but did not contain any human emotion.

It was also around this time that Dad began seesawing – in one letter he would say how impossible I was to live with, in the next he would come over all chauvinist about Cristiana. He called Mum to compare notes. 'Poor Clive seems to have certain problems in his home life and my heart bleeds for both of them,' he said. 'I mean, there can be no doubt that he cannot be the easiest of people to live with given his dedication to his work, and it surely needs a special type of mate to cope. Maybe if Cristiana can only get an independent career going, things may work out all right.'

Cristiana had troubles with that independent career. She had wanted to be an architect, but the five-year programme at Emory had dissuaded her. Then she worked for a company called Everything Is Gold which sold only silver. 'Someone is paying me for my time and that is *very* motivating,' she wrote to my mother. 'But my boss is very unpredictable, very unpleasant one moment, very nice the next.' She decided she wanted to be self-employed as an interior designer, and we set up Cristico. Her father bought the house across the street from us, and she spent long days trying to fix it up. It was lonely labour, bound eventually to destroy her soul, but she insisted on trying.

Cristiana was miserable. We did try marriage counselling. She chose the person, and the price – like Trailways bus tickets, it was only $10 per session. The therapist was apologetic about her lack of formal qualifications, but I respected her. She summed up our relationship quickly; I still have some of the notes of what we discussed. It was amicable, and Cristiana was protective of our relationship when we had those sessions, as if venting would be a betrayal.

One fact was not yet fully clear to either of us – that we were just very different people, and we had entered our marriage with optimism but without any health warnings.

There was an incident one night that made me walk out for good. I did not leave because of any fault in Cristiana, but because I encountered a part of me that I hated. I used to have loud dance parties – ABBA, Madonna, all-night affairs that would end with most of the alcohol sweated out in the Southern heat. This time the speakers blew, and someone managed to break a light switch. That night, when everyone had left much earlier than normal, we had a raging row. She said something taunting about my mother. I totally lost control of myself. Even as it was happening, I could not believe what I was doing. I was watching, aghast, from outside myself. I did manage to pull back at the last moment, but there it was, the awful term that Dad used – I was about to give her 'a little slap'. It didn't even slow Cristiana down, but it stopped me entirely. I was six-three, she was almost a foot smaller. I backed away at once.

In the morning, when I said I was going to leave, Cristiana asked me what I was so upset about. She insisted she had not even noticed that I had lost control of myself. I still find that hard to believe. Regardless, it was something I will never forget.

Up till that moment, I had taken part in intellectual discussions at law school about someone having an 'irresistible impulse'. I had not really stopped to think what it meant. I had been rigidly in control of myself since the fights I had been forced to endure at prep school. One of my colleagues coined a description of me: half-robot, half-machine. If being human meant losing control like that, I would rather be android.

Still, as I sat in a bar by myself, I had to wonder whether I had done worse things. I knew I was able to shut Cristiana out altogether. In the law we always talked about being a 'danger to self or others' in terms of physical injury, but maybe that was just wrong. Maybe I was actually more of a danger to her when I refused to engage emotionally with her at all.

Seeing my reflection in my beer glass, I saw failure. However naive I may have been, I had married her for better and for worse, yet it was all coming to an end after a very short time. Cristiana retreated to New York, while I stayed in Atlanta, but she did not want to split up. Though I knew I should stop, for months on end I spoke to her on the phone most nights, long calls that ended with her in tears.

'I do not understand Clive,' Cristiana wrote in a *cri de coeur* to my mother, as I got more distant on the phone. 'I do not understand how he went through separating so easily and how he now feels no pain.' Here, she was wrong. Those phone calls broke through my carapace; I still get flashbacks to the pain of them, true post-traumatic stress disorder. But eventually, I just had to dissociate again.

'Why did we part?' Cristiana pondered many years later. 'I did not want to play the part of the "first lady" any more than Hillary Clinton. It is not easy to live with a man like Clive.'

The defences I had constructed disintegrated momentarily in that one violent moment on Glenwood Avenue, and in response I built my wall still stronger.

What I should have looked to was the root cause of my loss of control, which was not Cristiana but rather my attempt to batten down all emotion forever. It was here, in the inability to understand how others see love, that Dad and I had most in common. I had always thought of myself as a romantic; as did he. He sat with a glass of brandy and wrote poems; I preferred gin when I penned my odes, and it had been my idea to marry on Valentine's Day.

Dad was obsessed with the idea of love, yet for him it was the romantic love of Don Quixote riding around the countryside rescuing a damsel at the end of his lance, without pausing to ask whether the dragon was her pet. Dad's definition of love – a yearning to feel the happiness and fulfilment of the loved one – was an intellectual concept. Gradually, Dad had fallen back when he found his 'definition' did not magically create some blanket around him. He became more alone. Indeed, he amended his 'definition' to provide that the yearning to feel the happiness of the loved one must begin by loving 'that little part of Creation called Self'.

Dad struggled even with this.

I also writhed in the wake of my divorce from Cristiana, wondering whether Dad was right when he said that I was impossible to live with. I sat outside the battered shack a friend lent me on the sand to the south of New Orleans, watching as the sun set over the Caribbean, incrementally replaced by the flickering flames of the drilling platforms burning off surplus gas. It was officially ranked one of the ten dirtiest beaches in the United States, which was what drew me to it. I could walk for miles without encountering anyone. I composed my latest sonnet, 'The Luxury of Loneliness'. I listed the compatibilities that would be necessary for anyone to get along with me, and my own antipathies that would render any relationship impossible.

I am told that love is not one emotion, and that it does not exist without anger and even hatred. If that is so, I live in a fortress protected from all such feelings. My irritation will rarely rise above frustration. Pain is repressed before the next sunrise. I just don't get the point of hatred. But I am not entirely sure I get love either. I should have come with Alain de Botton's health warning. So should Dad.

14

Larry Lonchar Finds Life's Meaning in Gambling

One turn of the wheel, and everything changes . . . What am I today? Zero. What can I be tomorrow? Tomorrow I may rise from the dead and start to live again!

Fyodor Dostoevsky, *The Gambler*

It had taken a long time, but two lives were rapidly converging: Larry Lonchar's and mine. In 1984, around the same time as I left law school to begin my battles in the Deep South, Larry's mother, Elsie, had just got herself sectioned again: after she divorced Milan Sr, she tried suicide. Gary Brown, the psychologist at Lakeview Hospital in Battle Creek, felt she appeared intellectually 'dull'. She had also been heavily medicated with Tofranil and Mellaril for anxiety for nine years.

'Why are you here?' Dr Brown asked. She described drinking one or two beers maybe twice a week, but he knew this was false, as she had a long history of unbridled alcoholism. She complained of insomnia when not taking her medication, as well as poor appetite and a lack of concentration – the stomach distress was, he concluded, entirely somatic. They were the classic signs of a clinical depression.

'Have you ever felt down?' he asked.

'Not me!' she insisted. 'I'm usually a happy-go-lucky individual.' She did admit that her husband had gambled and drunk all through their marriage, which she described as 'pure hell'. 'A lot of times we didn't have food in the house. I just stayed with him for the kids.' He used to beat the kids as well as the patient. 'He beat me up once and left me for dead. After that time was when I left him.'

Overall, she insisted, she had maintained a good relationship with her children, though she was quite concerned about Larry, her son who was again in prison. He had been incarcerated on three occasions. He would get out for two or three months, then do something to go back inside.

Elsie was not much of a historian of her own history. She omitted the drunken brawls that happened almost every evening, and the grunting sex in the basement as she graduated from affairs to prostituting herself. I doubt the doctor knew anything of the impact of this on young Larry Lonchar. Larry was not within the ambit of his responsibility – or anyone else's.

Elsie went back to the ward, where she tended to huddle near the television most of the time, unless she was huddling against the Michigan winter outside, sucking hard on a cigarette. Meanwhile, Brown dictated the report for his supervisor: 'Mrs Lonchar has a Verbal IQ 77, Performance IQ 75 and a Full Scale IQ of 75, placing this patient's current intellectual functioning in the borderline mentally deficient range. The Machover Drawings are frankly grotesque. We see representations of psychosexual confusion and mixed identification, severe deterioration in ego boundaries, distorted self-image, immaturity, and dependency. One would judge these the productions of an individual suffering from organicity [brain damage] and psychosis.'

Brown had done some other tests. 'In the Rorschach protocol we see repeated signs of immaturity, underlying feelings of inadequacy, a schizoid orientation in interpersonal relationships, and regression. One suspects that this patient feels that her emotional supports have weakened over the years. There are hints of a possible schizophrenic process. For example, she sees "a big dark tree – it's bad – it's deteriorated". There are periodic signs of paranoia.'

The psychologist concluded: 'Her overall psychometric evidence reveals a chronic depression, organic brain syndrome and at the very least a severe schizoid personality with hypochondriacal features. One might speculate that this patient's somatic complaints may act as a first line of defense against a florid outcropping of psychosis. I would recommend continued hospitalization and supportive psychotherapy.'

What did all these tests actually say about who Elsie was, and – more importantly – about how her life might be made more satisfying? So often, as Larry would soon find out, a psychologist has too little time to get to know the patient, and the tests were a substitute for the hours, days and weeks that might allow for proper help.

What about Larry, then? 'Although it may seem to be a contradiction in terms, gambling is as spiritual as praying,' writes anthropologist Kathryn Gabriel. 'Both activities seek divine affirmation and reversal of fortune. In other words, the gambler, unbeknownst to himself, is looking for divinity. Sure, on the surface he is seeking economic fortune, but he is also seeking a personal transformation, for that feeling of invincibility and liberation, even if only in the moment of exhilaration.'

For Larry, gambling, if not divine, defined his ego. Every time he laid a card down, he made a decision, a choice that coloured in the frail sketch of his life. Like boarding school had done for me, prison did not leave much room for individual choices in the framing of his day. Rules governed most of his moves. Gambling was technically illegal in Michigan's penitentiary system, but the authorities turned Nelson's blind eye. For Larry it was both work and play: his mother was in the asylum, so he had nobody on the outside who would keep him in commissary. His needs were modest, for his limited luxuries were splash-on cologne for his self-esteem, and junk-food supplements to the prison cuisine.

Larry became an accomplished card player, and he soon

graduated to the premier division of poker in his institution, where there was no certainty of winning or losing. Indeed, certainty would have been nihilism. In the Michigan Department of Corrections, he won more than he lost, and he could always pay his debts on time. If he was on a losing streak, he could get credit up to a certain limit; if he looked to be approaching his maximum, he could make up some of his losses in the lower-stakes games among the lesser players.

Yet betting a few dollars is not an epitaph. Ultimately, a committed gambler must be prepared to stake, and potentially lose, everything. Perhaps he will even stake his life. (Nevada, long the bastion of legalised gambling, has a suicide rate more than double the national average.)

As Larry emerged from prison in Michigan, on parole after an eight-year stretch for robbery, he decided that neither his mother nor his home state had much to offer him, so he transferred to Georgia where his sister now lived. However, the Georgia parole authorities left him little room for life either. He was required to hold down a job paying $165 for a forty-hour week. Counting out dollar bills on his kitchen table after the authorities had garnished a percentage to pay his victim restitution, and more to pay his supervision fee, he barely had enough to pay for his tiny apartment and eat. But if he remained patient for a few years, the authorities promised, he would be off parole. One day perhaps he would get married, and be free to spend the rest of his life hoping that his children would do better.

Because gambling had given Larry some liberty in prison, he decided to gamble again now in the hope that he might truly become free. He started small, with legal giveaways advertised in *Contest Newsletter*, a weekly magazine where advertisers promised a range of prizes for taking part in different sweepstakes. His dreamworld was littered across the carpet of his flat.

'Lauren Hyde is one of the six regional winners,' boasted that month's 'Winformation' column. 'Actually, Pumpkin her cat is the winner in the Meow Off Sweepstakes. We hope she claws her way right to the top.' Pumpkin was more fortunate than Larry, who had been tempted by the Häagen-Dazs Life's Rich Rewards Sweepstakes. First prize was a $35,000 Jaguar XJ6. Larry lost. He never hit the McKenzie's Bakery Bingo or the Piggly-Wiggly Power Hour either.

As Larry faced his empty mailbox, he knew he had to graduate. He had his own copy of John Fisher's book, *Never Give a Sucker an Even Break: Tricks and Bets You Can't Lose*, but Larry had to identify the suckers while they tried to do the same to him. Gambling was not legal in Georgia in the mid-1980s either, which meant there was a central paradox: there was no granny-state rule capping the stakes, so illegal gambling dens could offer a bet without seeing any money upfront, since they could collect at the end of a snub-nosed revolver if they had to. Larry was a gambling addict; Wayne Smith was a small-time crook who liked to boast that he was tied to the Mob. He ran his gambling from an apartment in DeKalb County, just outside Atlanta, and allowed almost unlimited credit.

Larry's initials (LL) and telephone number – 991-0071 – appeared for the first time on the sixth page of Smith's betting book. The wagers made by punters each day were recorded in scribbled lists, beside Smith's shorthand identifier, with no last names. Years later, as I plotted the unfolding chart of Larry's life, I felt an increasing nausea. He was a good card player, where skill supplemented chance. In prison his good fortune – perhaps a full house – had been complemented by an understanding of the statistics, and a talent for judging the nervous mannerisms of his opponents. Now Larry turned to bets based on the foibles of a football team. The odds – the 'line' – were dictated by Wayne Smith. Larry had to do more than pick the winning team. Since one team would inevitably be the favourite, it would be handicapped by the spread – if the bet was Harvard over Yale by at least fourteen points, he would win if the final scoreline was 34–20, but lose if Harvard prevailed 34–21.

When I understood this, I thought Larry had descended into madness. This was not a game of skill; it was worse than horses on the track. In the end, Larry was diving into the same cesspit that had bankrupted Dad. 'LL' debuted in Smith's book of bets on a Saturday. That day, someone going by the initials JT won $400 and lost $110, coming out $290 ahead; BP placed twelve bets for a total of $1,730, and won $170 overall; the day was sour for 'Mike' who lost $670. Larry planned to win big and get his life on track. His largest bet was an astounding $660 on my alma mater, the University of North Carolina, who were heavily favoured to beat Wake Forest, an Atlantic Coast Conference rival. Larry bet them to win on a spread of nine and a half points. I felt ill at the idea of Larry staking more than a month's income on UNC. I had witnessed the frailty of their football team in several losing games and could not remember a time when they had ever won by as many as ten points.

The weekend was a catastrophe. UNC were the first to betray him. They did not simply fail to win by a large enough margin – the final score was UNC 10, Wake Forest 21. Larry would have been watching on television, and must have known his $660 was gone fifteen minutes into the game. He backed eight other colleges that day, and every one failed him. At the end of the day, Larry's win column was vacant and his loss column totalled $3,410. If he did not eat, if he went homeless, if he refused to pay taxes and if he did not pay his parole officer, it would still take Larry five months to pay the cost of one afternoon of real living.

I continued to chart Larry's progress. After his first foray into Smith's betting book, I thought he might pull back in horror. But Larry saw there was no point betting if he could not get back at least to even. Instead of shrinking towards his income, his bets burgeoned. He did do better the second weekend, coming out $2,090 ahead, and this cut his debt to $1,320. That was the last time he ever won more than he lost.

In week three, while most of the others in Smith's book posted modest wins, Larry lost $1,900. Soon, the page with Larry's initials reflected a total debt of $10,290. At the weekend, then, he bet a staggering total of $11,400. He must have cheered when the first teams won by wide margins. He was up by $3,390. Yet by the end of the day, six weeks in, he owed $14,910. The scale of his losses may have seemed unreal to begin with, little more than Monopoly money, but this was Smith's business, and his pleasure lay in collecting his debts. Smith made it clear that if Larry did not start paying, the enforcers would be called in.

'It's normal. He'd have to do it to me,' Larry later told me, his voice phlegmatically matter-of-fact. 'He'd have no choice.'

The desperation that had led Larry to up the ante each week now had the dangerous odour of fear. The first visit from Smith's collection agents would not prove fatal, but could be very painful. Larry did not have many options. He could rob a few convenience stores, but it would take several heists to make a dent in his debt. Or he could try to find another way.

The prosecution later developed a theory: Larry considered his options, they decided, and in October 1986 elected to launch a pre-emptive strike against his creditor.

15

A Senseless Triple Murder

Knowing once more the whitehot joy
Of taking human life

Lieutenant Colonel George S. Patton,
'Peace – November 11, 1918'

DeKalb County was less than a mile from my house on Glenwood Avenue. I had no idea who Larry Lonchar was when the tragedy unfolded – any more than he did me. If the prosecution was correct, Larry's plan was ingenious, and involved nobody getting hurt. If Fortune had robbed Larry of his anticipated winnings, then he was here to seize them back. He and his confederates would pose as FBI agents, playing on the fact that the gambling den was illegal. They would knock on the door of Wayne Smith's condo and conduct the arrest. They would then be able to search the flat for all the money Smith had taken betting. Thousands of dollars in bank deposits could not be honestly explained, so it was likely that cash would be lying around before it could be laundered somehow.

Under the prosecution theory, Larry would have his meal ticket out of Georgia, and enough money to go on the run from the parole authorities. His prior crimes were not of a type that would put him on the FBI's Most Wanted list, and robbing a criminal gambling den would hardly up the ante: his odds of evading capture were certainly better than trying to pull off a string of armed robberies.

If this was truly the plan, it went awry from the start. According to the prosecution's theory, Larry stood slightly to one side of the front door, wearing a long raincoat and a fedora hat. He knocked. Wayne Smith recognised him, and allowed him into the front room. This was the first of many points where the prosecution, preparing the case for trial, would later be unsure. They knew that he was accompanied into the room by at least one other person, Mitchell (Mitch) Wells, but they strongly suspected that a third person was also present. Who might that have been?

Larry supposedly showed a badge.

'I'm Special Agent Larry Lonchar of the FBI,' the prosecution theorised him saying. They had brought only two sets of handcuffs. From his visits there over the past six weeks, Larry knew Wayne would often be alone, with just a possibility that his son Steve would be there to help him. So what was the occasion? Why were there four people? Wayne was in the living room with his girlfriend, Margaret Sweat, and Steve. Wayne said a second son, Charles, was in the bedroom.

'It's been a sting operation, on your illegal gambling,' the prosecutors imagined Larry telling the shocked Smiths as he pulled out the cuffs. 'You two' – indicating Wayne and Steve – 'are under arrest.' He sent Margaret into a different bedroom from Charles, to get her out of the way. Soon, though, Charles was the last one alive. He would be the only witness, but he saw and heard little. He was lying on a bed as he heard the voices, then four or five shots from the living room. Before he had time to move, a man he later identified as Mitch Wells came in and shot him once in the back, and once – fortunately just a graze – aimed at the head. He pretended to be dead, listening to the intruders as they ransacked the house.

After a while, fearing that he would bleed to death, Charles crawled to the telephone to call for help. As he picked up the phone, he heard Margaret Sweat's voice speaking on the other handset. It was standard for the emergency call to be tape-recorded – less standard to record a death, as happened this time. It was dramatic evidence when it was later played for the jurors.

'DeKalb Emergency,' the emergency operator answered.

'Police?' said Margaret.

'What address?' the operator asked, but Margaret's answer was too faint to be heard. 'What's the problem?'

'Everybody's been shot,' she said.

'Who's been shot?' the operator asked.

Lying in her own blood, Margaret could not have known the extent of the carnage around her. 'Me . . . and . . .' she replied uncertainly.

'With a gun?' the operator asked, sounding rather stupid when the tape was played later.

'Yes.'

'Who did it?'

'I don't know.'

'Is that a house or an apartment?'

'It's a condominium.'

'OK. Now you say everybody's been shot, I already got you help on the way.' The operator tried to comfort her, having dispatched patrol vehicles and an ambulance to the scene. 'But when you say everybody's been shot, how many?'

'Uh, me.' Margaret was unable to see the corpses of her boyfriend and his elder son.

'Where are you shot at?'

'In the living room – I've crawled to the phone.'

'I mean what part of your body, ma'am.'

'I think my stomach . . .' she said. In shock, she did not know where her wound was, or that it was far from fatal.

At that moment she heard the door open again. 'They're coming back in . . . please . . .' Again, her voice became inaudibly faint.

'Who did it?' The operator did not know that he was about to hear her being killed. 'Give me a description of them!'

'Why are you doing this?' Margaret moved to try to protect herself from the second attack. 'Please . . . [inaudible] . . . Please! . . . Please! . . . I don't even know your name! . . . Please . . . please . . . Larry . . . I don't even know your name . . .'

The operator listened as Margaret seemed to deny knowing the name she had just spoken. Was this evidence against Larry, as the prosecution would argue? Or was this a hint to the defence lawyer? Was there an alternative explanation for everything?

The call went silent. The assailant had perhaps pulled the phone wire from the wall. Charles crawled into the living room just in time to see a man in a trench coat run out – who he would describe as inconsistent with Larry's build. When the police arrived, they rushed Charles to the hospital. There was no saving the other three. Wayne and Steve had each been shot first in the chest, then the back and the head. Margaret Sweat had been shot once in the shoulder, then stabbed several times in the neck and the chest.

The prosecution theorised that Larry had come back in and finished her off with a knife. Larry's cousin Johnny 'Dougie' McLiechey testified against him at trial. According to him, Larry had come by the house looking for Wells on his way out of town. 'I couldn't kill the bitch,' Larry had said, according to his cousin, himself on parole for bank robbery. Again, the words were fatally ambiguous, assuming that Larry's cousin repeated them accurately. Had he been trying to do it, or was he claiming he could never have done it?

McLiechey had driven him to Chattanooga, where Larry caught a plane to Texas. The police put pressure on McLiechey to inculpate his cousin, threatening him with prosecution as an accessory. The police then had him wire Larry some money to a Western Union in Mission, Texas. It was a set-up. When he saw what was happening, Larry ran towards the arresting officer.

'Shoot me!' he shouted. 'Shoot me!'

Shortly after his arrest, an officer tried to interrogate him.

'It's pointless to tell anyone what happened, I just want to get the trial over with and die,' Larry said, pausing for a moment. 'You can do me one favour, though.'

The detective nodded for him to carry on.

'You could ask my mother to buy a cemetery plot, if you wouldn't mind.' For most of the time I knew him, Larry was scrupulously polite.

Larry was suicidal. That was nothing new. His parole officer, Amber Watson, had been counselling him long before the triple murder. Now he had plenty of reason to be in a dark place: he was thirty-five, he had gone nowhere in life, and he was going to die in prison – either in the chair or thirty years down the line. And he was in Georgia, a state he hated; everything about it was redneck and regressive.

Larry's case was to be held in Decatur, a liberal satellite town to Georgia's state capital, Atlanta. The trial judge, Robert Castellani, was in his early forties, tall, stooped and slightly balding. He had been an Assistant Attorney General, then a federal magistrate and now, for the past two years, an elected trial judge. He was deeply religious and he understood something about the dangers of power, as his father had fled Fascism in Italy. I already knew him slightly since he appeared at some of the criminal defence events to balance out the expected attendance at prosecutor meetings. He seemed to care for those who came before him – a platinum rarity in a world where most elected judges were clambering over the bodies of people they sentenced to death, seeking the golden snitch of higher judicial office.

Castellani immediately appointed counsel to represent Larry – Cal Leipold, a committed defence lawyer, although without experience in death penalty defence. The United States Supreme Court had ruled in 1985, in *Ake* v. *Oklahoma*, that a capital defendant had the right to a mental health evaluation where appropriate. Judge Castellani let Leipold have two experts to assess Larry.

Working out how to present someone to twelve people making a life-and-death decision is a challenging and complicated process. As I got somewhat better at the job, I would average three years in preparing for a capital trial, by which time I knew my client better than he knew himself. The job of the mental health practitioner in a capital case should be the ultimate challenge: what brought this person from the cradle, with all that human potential, to this point, sitting before a jury who could decide when they would go to their grave?

However, market forces were at work then and now – in the late 1980s, the defence expert might be limited to $500 or $1,000 for a 'full' evaluation and testimony. This often meant that experts spent only a couple of hours in an interview. At best, they would have a *Reader's Digest* edition of a life, perhaps only from the defendant; it was rare for them to talk to family members. For any documentation of the defendant's background, they were in the hands of the lawyers, who ranged from the overworked and inexperienced local public defender to unfunded messianic devotees like me.

For all our law school debates, in the Deep South a verdict of 'not guilty by reason of insanity' in a capital trial was rarer than a happy prison population – I have never had such a result in all the cases I have done. In order to vote NGBRI a jury must think the person on trial really killed someone in a dreadful way and was totally deranged at the time. Inevitably they worry that some doctor will let the defendant out of hospital and there will be nothing to stop him or her doing it again.

More relevant, then, the defence must identify something in mitigation of a terrible crime. There are many ways that the notion of premeditation might be diminished: jurors might understand the impact that drinking or taking drugs has on rational planning; most people could empathise with provocation and loss of control (even I did, by this point); perhaps the gun went off once, in the moment, but at least the accused didn't keep pumping the victim full of lead.

Then there is a spectrum of 'mental disorders' that might be taken into account, and this is where the battle of the penalty-phase experts normally takes place. Here, the debate can easily be lost in the fog of lawfare. 'Experts' tend to fall back on the comfortable labels in the *DSM*, with its broad classifications and magical medical jargon. Thus, a defendant might have a horrific history of abuse: in the hands of the defence expert, this means that he could not control his explosive disorder. In the hands of a prosecution expert, the diagnosis will be anti-social personality disorder (ASPD) – the accused is someone with no conscience who will kill again.

Prosecutors are inordinately fond of ASPD, which is purportedly identified by a long-term pattern of disregard for the rights of others – a selfish desire to get what you can for yourself. To qualify, according to the *DSM*, a person must exhibit *either* 'self-esteem derived from personal gain, power, or pleasure' *or* 'goal-setting based on personal gratification' – this probably included the majority of my colleagues at Columbia Law School who wanted to be well-heeled lawyers. Next, one might show a 'lack of concern for the feelings, needs, or suffering of others'. At the age of seven, when asked in class what it meant to be a Conservative, my son said, 'they don't like to share'. The 'pathological personality traits' of ASPD include the 'use of subterfuge to influence or control others or the use of seduction, charm, glibness, or ingratiation to achieve one's ends'. There are various politicians who fit this bill.

Another refuge of the mental health scoundrel are the psychological tests, such as those given earlier to Elsie Lonchar. Building a rapport with the patient over days and weeks takes far too long when you are asked to do a fly-by psychological evaluation. Too often, experts substitute in a Rorschach ink-blot test, a Draw-a-Person test and a Minnesota Multiphasic Personality Inventory (MMPI). Perhaps unsurprisingly, a study in California identified three groups of people who appear to be sociopathic on the MMPI: doctors, lawyers and murderers. None of the three career paths, as practised in the US, requires generosity of spirit. To me, this suggests certain lessons: one, that none of this necessarily means much; two, that such a 'diagnosis' tells us little about how we can help someone adapt to society – or how society can adapt to allow the individual to live with us.

With Larry Lonchar, the hired experts would have to evaluate whether there were any factors that might mitigate his sentence from death to life in prison.

Leipold chose two experts: Randi Most, PhD, was a psychologist who did a pre-trial evaluation of Larry; Dr Lloyd Baccus was the consulting psychiatrist. However, Leipold had a very limited budget.

When I looked her up later, I found Dr Most's website to be very American. One section listed the accepted forms of payment; another had the form contract setting her fee at $125–150 an hour; a third was devoted entirely to Dusty, noting the regrettable death of a 'Bedlington terrier certified through Therapy Dogs International . . . a part of Dr Most's practice since she was a puppy. Dusty welcomed people to the office and did her best to ensure that everyone was feeling calm and relaxed. Dusty also appeared on TV's *Animal Planet*. Dusty will be missed by all.'

Sadly, Dusty was not there for Larry Lonchar's evaluation; he liked animals, and would have related to the dog. He did not trust Dr Most. His review of her to me years later was anodyne – which, in Larry's vocabulary, was not good. Some online reviews of her practice were positive, others not.

She met with Larry and pulled out her various tests. Larry had no motive to cooperate – he was suicidal and wanted to die. This should have been a difficult evaluation where she would have to find a way to dissolve his self-destruction. She did not do this.

'Mr Lonchar presented as a slim, sandy-haired male who

looked his stated age,' she wrote in her report. 'He was quite reluctant to undergo testing, indicating that he was "not insane" and that no one could help him.' She therefore concluded that he had 'provided no valid data from which to draw inferences concerning his personality dynamics'. She did note that he was depressed and hopeless, which hardly required a PhD. Her evaluation told us absolutely nothing.

Dr Baccus filed his own report on Larry Lonchar soon after. I had already come across him. Born on Christmas Day 1939, he was a glib chap who I found too concerned about the finances of his office. He met with Larry just once. He knew Larry had been in prison (that was in all the records). He knew Larry was charged with a senseless triple murder. Larry was far too loyal to his family to tell the doctor about his chaotic background.

'Mr Lonchar presents with a history consistent with a diagnosis of antisocial personality disorder,' he concluded. 'There is no indication of the presence of a psychiatric disorder of such a nature as to interfere with his capacity to conform his conduct to the law at the time of the alleged offenses. Thank you for this opportunity to interview this interesting individual.'

Dr Baccus, too, was simply throwing Larry away. Translated into English, he was saying that Larry knew right from wrong, and if he had committed this crime it was because he was essentially a sociopath, someone who would not be too troubled by murder.

At this time I had not yet met Larry. When I did, I would represent him – and get to know him – for over eight years. It can safely be said that Dr Baccus had no idea what he was talking about.

Larry initially insisted that he wanted the death penalty without a trial.

'I told Lonchar who I was and that I wanted to give him an opportunity to tell his side of the story,' said Detective Charles

Buis, the DeKalb County officer with primary responsibility for the case. 'Lonchar said that we both knew that would be a waste of time, that we had enough on him to put him in the electric chair, and that he had come back to Georgia to die. I asked him what he meant, and he said that he wasn't going to put his family and the victims' families through a trial, that he was going to plead guilty and die in the chair. Also that if they didn't give him the electric chair, he would kill himself.'

Despite his initial promise to the detective, Larry found he was stymied by the law. Even though there were three dead victims, the state suggested to Leipold that if Larry pled guilty they would not seek the death penalty – he would then automatically be sentenced to life imprisonment, the long path towards a desert before him. Still, Larry figured out that he could force them to go through a trial, and get the jury to kill him. He had never had the courage to end it all, but he could still make someone else do it for him.

Larry's trial was approaching. There was clearly more to the story than the prosecution originally believed and a careful prosecutor would have been worried. The prosecution's fingerprint technician determined that the only print found on the handcuffs that had been used to restrain two of the victims belonged to Mitch Wells. The surviving eyewitness, Charles 'Rick' Smith, identified Wells as the one who had pulled the trigger on him. The ballistics expert said that all the bullets fired at all four victims came out of the same gun – Wells's weapon. Larry's cousin would say what the prosecution wanted, but his testimony that Larry said 'I couldn't kill the bitch' was ambiguous, and everyone mistrusts a snitch. The dramatic 911 tape, leading up to and during Margaret Sweat's death, was also opaque. Charles glimpsed her killer and described a third person, taller than Larry. In addition to the blood of the victim, Margaret Sweat, there was blood from an unknown person on the knife – not Wells's, not Larry's; it is hard to stab someone repeatedly without the knife slipping and damaging oneself, and it is not unusual to find the assailant's blood intermixed with the victim's.

'What difference would it make if I did tell the whole truth?' Larry dolefully demanded of Cal Leipold. 'I was present, there's no getting round that. They say I planned a robbery, so under Georgia law I'm guilty of murder even if someone else actually pulled the trigger.'

Leipold tried to talk him round. If he had not done the actual killing, he could not be sentenced to death. Larry had an extensive and exemplary prison record. A key question for a capital juror is: *Why do we need to kill him? If he is going to stay in prison forever, behaving well, we do not need to execute him.* With a relatively liberal DeKalb County jury, it would not have been difficult to avoid the death penalty.

'Death?' Larry exclaimed dismissively. 'What do I care about death? What's worse, three times a life sentence in some Georgia prison, or death? Same thing, ain't it? I been dying a long time now . . .' His voice trailed off.

Larry stewed in his jail cell, working on other ways to make a bad situation worse. He decided that he did not even want to be at his trial. In a capital case, this was unprecedented. The law said that Larry had an absolute right to be present while his fate was decided. Cal Leipold was horrified; the first rule in defending someone in a capital trial is to humanise them. Judge Robert Castellani asked Larry to state his position on the record. Why did he want to be out of the room the whole time?

'I just repeat the way I feel, you know,' Larry said, adamant. 'My presence is irrelevant. And like I say, I haven't been assisting my attorney and I am not going to start assisting him.'

'There's a tightrope there that you're walking,' Assistant DA Jim Richter, the lead prosecutor, told the judge. 'I think you should avoid it.' He thought the judge should make Larry attend the whole trial. So did Cal Leipold, who was desperate to have his client present.

Judge Castellani pondered the dilemma. Ultimately, he announced that Larry would be allowed to sit in his cell for much of the trial and only come into court when he had to be identified by a witness.

An Irish patriot once commented on the British efforts to see him hanged: 'They tried me *in absentia*. They sentenced me to death *in absentia*. They can damned well execute me *in absentia*.' American law is also of the view that the defendant must be present throughout proceedings, and there were various cases directly on point from the Eleventh Circuit Court of Appeals, the federal court that had jurisdiction over the state of Georgia. If the client is not disruptive, he cannot be excluded; even if he makes a scene, the judge is required to take gradual steps towards shackling and gagging him, but the client can never be removed from the courtroom. If he were, any verdict is bound to be reversed on appeal. Judge Castellani had to know this was legal quicksand.

If there was one way to try to ensure that a death sentence imposed on Larry in 1987 would be reversed in 1997 or 2007, it was for the state trial judge to read a written opinion by a federal court and then do precisely the opposite. I later wondered whether Judge Castellani just didn't want a death sentence on his conscience.

The trial began, and Larry sat in his cell for most of it. At the end, the jurors debated for two hours, without having heard a defence. He was convicted of three counts of murder. When it came to the penalty phase, again Larry refused to be present. The prosecution introduced his prior convictions for robbery in Michigan. Larry's father, Milan, did take the stand, against his son's wishes. He felt guilty that he had done little for his son in the previous thirty-five years, so now he felt compelled to speak. He gave only a very edited version of the nightmare of

Larry's Battle Creek childhood. 'I'd love to have my son live,' he said, pleadingly, to the jury.

'I'd like to see my brother and father too,' muttered Charles Smith, audibly, from the front row of the audience.

Most capital trials I have done have involved two or three days of evidence for life. Leipold did not have much to work with, but he argued as best he could. He begged for mercy. 'Don't take this man's life,' he said in closing. 'Put him in the prison system for the rest of his life, but don't take his life.'

There was a brief break before the prosecution gave the final demand for death. 'Miss Sweat didn't have anybody else to beg for her life,' said Richter when his turn came. 'She begged him herself. This was a cold-blooded, ruthless execution that violates every kind of rule that we hold dear in our society.' For half an hour he detailed why they should send Larry to the electric chair. 'The world is not going to miss Larry Lonchar,' he said at the climax of his argument. 'The world would be better off without him here.'

I have sat through such arguments in court many times. Can there be a more deranged and hate-filled speech than a prosecutor's argument that a fellow human being is so worthless that he or she should be taken out and ceremonially murdered? Perhaps Larry was fortunate to miss it.

Even without much of a case before them, the jurors struggled. They started debating on Thursday; all day Friday they worked on. At 10.30 that night, Judge Castellani sent them back to the motel, telling them they would resume the next morning. Only when they had exhausted everything they had to say, and exhausted the jurors who resisted death, did they come back with their verdict on the Saturday afternoon.

It was death by electrocution.

Judge Castellani ordered the verdict sealed because he did not want to taint Mitch Wells's trial, due to start on Monday. Wells, though, told his lawyers to get over to the prosecution office and accept the outstanding offer of life – an offer that Larry could easily have got himself. After all, Charles Smith was going to come into court, take the witness stand, and point directly at Wells as the one who almost killed him. There was no ambiguity in his case.

Judge Castellani did not enjoy what he had to do. He read out his order.

'It is considered, ordered and adjudged that within a time period commencing at noon on the 10th day of August, and ending at noon on the 16th day of August . . . the defendant Larry Grant Lonchar shall be executed by the Department of Corrections . . . all in accordance with the law of Georgia. And may God have mercy on your soul.'

He meant the part about mercy. But Larry finally had what he said he wanted.

16

The Bank Manager and
the Build-up to the Libel

Insanity is hereditary – you get it from your children.

Sam Levenson

It was my birthday, and I opened the bowling for the Metro-politan Cricket Club (MCC) against the Tropical Cricket Club (TCC). We were playing on a matting wicket in the Atlanta suburbs. The captain of the MCC was Conrad Hunte, former vice captain of the West Indies. After scoring 260 against Pakistan in a partnership of 446 with Gary Sobers (who went on to make 365), he now found himself surrounded by dreadful amateurs like me. He was an immoderately modest man who always encouraged us when he might have complained. The TCC had three former international players and I dropped Desmond Lewis, the former West Indies keeper, third ball for nought off my own bowling. We could not afford that kind of thing. Their team, vulnerable at the start of the innings when they were sober, became unstoppable when they loosened up over a few slugs of rum.

Dad was in Spain. His mood was oscillating. Some of the time he saw no hope; sometimes the future of the known world rested on his latest project, SAPPSA (I never could get a straight answer out of him about what the acronym stood for). Spiralling upwards, he announced he was distributing the (imaginary) shares in SAPPSA – Mary and I were to receive two hundred, twice as many as Mark, for he was currently in the doghouse for a perceived slight. On a whim, Dad's old private school, the Perse, got two hundred too, and even the local car-hire centre and the Ronda police were to get fifty each. He sent his 'Plan for the Future of Ronda Real' to the local council: *Real* meant 'Royal' in this context, rather than bona fide. There was to be a new university there, and a large horse complex. He detailed how the town management was currently a 'disgrace', so it was fortunate he two-finger-typed the plan in English, a language I hoped they might not understand.

He also sent his Ronda plans to King Juan Carlos. Unfortunately, rather than ignoring him, the king's secretary replied with a polite form letter, so Dad thought his university was as good as built. He therefore sent a long epistle to Queen Elizabeth about the project, soliciting her support in an august collaboration over the sport of queens. At the time, I was busy and paid no attention to his letters. Later, I puzzled over what it all meant. It was lazy simply to dismiss this as 'Dad is mad'. Yes, it was grandiose in a way that was totally unrealistic. Sometimes I am guilty of that myself: I once got excited about an idea I had for restructuring the housing market in Britain and spent much of the night writing it up. I have often pondered how I might redraft a socialist agenda in a way to make equality a reality.

Meanwhile, aside from the rude tone, which hinted at an Asperger's- or autistic-style failure to appreciate the norms of society, Dad's letters did nobody any harm. They did illustrate how far afield he was, sitting on the balcony of his Marbella apartment. He wrote separately to me asking me to chase up getting him six hundred horses, each of a value up to £30,000. Since this reflected an investment of around £18 million, I was not in a position immediately to comply. While one view of these plans is that they were simply folly, another is that they were a cry for help. He wanted interaction with those who had not, yet, completely abandoned him. Sadly, he got none from me.

Because all of us wrote him off as mad, Dad was driven further along the promontory of loneliness. Previously, when he was full of energy, he had enjoyed a fair amount of money; now he had none to blow on grandiose plans. He had nowhere to turn his frustrated energies but upon those closest to him. None of us was quite prepared for it. He sent a series of vitriolic letters to Mum, accusing her of imaginary affairs in the early days of their marriage, such that some variation on the postman was father to Mark, Mary and me. He sent two of Auntie Jean's letters back to her, heavily annotated in red. 'Your last two letters are so appalling – even by your standards of uncaring and utter stupidity that I feel bound to return them!' he wrote. In between insulting her, he mentioned that he had just bought a *finca* (a farm of sorts) worth at least £3 million for only £550,000 and he expected later the same day to sell off about a quarter of it to pay for the rest. This was all fantasy. Nobody had been unwise enough to sell him anything beyond, perhaps, some tapas.

Dad then wrote to Mary. He wanted to borrow £5,000 on the flat we had bought for him with money generously put in trust by Auntie Jean. Short on a few pesetas, let alone imaginary millions, he wanted money with which to create a business. His first letter dressed it up well – the kitchen needed repairs, and he would get it done cheaply. Gradually, as he forgot his original pitch, his other goals emerged in increasingly angry letters: if he was going to achieve SAPPSA's vitally important goals at Ronda University, it was no good if he did not have the kind of equipment he needed for a proper office, like a fax and a telex.

He knew better than to mention what he really wanted, which was a telephone – this was not the mobile phone of today, with a tariff and EU rules cutting back the costs. One of the original debts he had acquired in bankruptcy had been hundreds of pounds to the telephone company. My own phone-phobia derived in large part from the way he would ruin a holiday by swerving towards a phone box at any moment to make an 'important' call. But he knew that the fax would have a line, so he could make all the phone calls he wanted.

Mary was the one currently in the UK, and it was her misfortune that she was acting as spokesperson for the three of us. Certainly we were not going to agree to him borrowing on the apartment, as he would then not repay the loan, the bank would foreclose, and we would be another home down with nowhere to put him. Mary was caught in the normal double bind: if she told him that we just did not trust his plans ever to come to anything, he would turn on her. If she did not give a reason for refusing the money, she would be chastised for being a stupid and illogical woman. She tried to turn his request back on him – perhaps he would be kind enough to earn the money himself for any improvements he wanted to make on the place, since we were at the extent of our finances in paying for it, as well as the small monthly subsidy we were sending him.

'I have just had a letter from poor Mary,' Dad wrote to Mum, 'which, I am sure she will agree, reads as though it has been written by an ill-mannered bank manager! I have sent it back to her. You have never attached a great deal of importance to good manners but I believe that they are of paramount importance to the smooth functioning of society and it is for this reason that I love living here in Andalusia where manners are so very, very good.'

The battle against Mary-the-Bank-Manager would run for months in letters that became increasingly vituperative, and would ultimately end only when I committed my own cardinal sin.

17

Is Religion an Indicator of Psychosis?

I disapprove of what you say, but I will defend to the death your right to say it.

Evelyn Beatrice Hall

In between missives about Mary, Dad wrote a spate of letters to the Archbishop of Canterbury and a number of bishops. 'I have decided that I was absolutely correct in 1963 to identify Paul as the cause of all the problems with the Church,' he began. 'I intend to spend some time in the next few years redefining Christ's message in modern terminology.' His latest monograph was titled *Resurrection or Reincarnation – a Study of Relative Efficiency*. When I first received my copy, I glanced over it. Sometimes, there was a good deal of sense in what Dad referred to as his 'little books', but on this occasion there was more that made me concerned about him. His emerging obsession with reincarnation struck me as a fatuous desire for another go after the mess he had made of this tenure on the planet. I did not worry enough, though. I was just too busy with my own life.

If I thought Dad's focus was a reflection of what might be called a 'mental disorder', then I sometimes felt surrounded by similar anomalies in the Deep South. Along with a couple of local public defenders, I was representing Willie Gamble in his capital murder trial at the time. Trials are far more complicated than appeals. I was very inexperienced, and I should not have been trusted with much more than trying a speeding offence at that point, but it was already my second jury trial where the death penalty was at issue. Willie lived in deep rural Georgia, not too far from Reidsville, home of the Georgia State Prison. He was charged with killing the wife and son of a prominent optometrist in Swainsboro.

I liked Willie from the moment I met him, and fairly soon I found it difficult to see how he could have come to have committed a double murder that had the white community in the mood for a lynching. He was a diminutive young black man, who shrank even further as I talked to him in the Emanuel County Jail. His mother was a gentle, religious woman. There was little escaping the fact that he had committed the act. He had done yard work for the victims, but while there were obvious racial divisions – Willie was clearly a 'coloured boy' to them – it was hard to understand his motive for murder.

Willie insisted that he had acted in self-defence: the victims had put a hex on him.

He was guileless. When he first said this, I barely suppressed a snigger. For me at the time, the word 'voodoo' conjured up Baron Samedi in the James Bond film *Live and Let Die*: a half-naked Haitian man, with his half-painted face, burning tarot cards while Mr Big interrogates Solitaire. The idea that a double homicide could have been caused by voodoo felt like a work of fiction.

Willie was deadly serious.

As with so many people I have represented, I learned a great deal from Willie. When I began to look into voodoo, I encountered new realities. Among the Tupinambá people, battle-hardened men died from fright when cursed by the witch doctor. Other famous cases of 'voodoo death' included the Maori woman who died because she ate an apple that she believed to be subject to a taboo, and the Aboriginal Australian men who died when they had a bone pointed at them. Willie was insisting that his actions were justified by self-defence – the victims were trying to kill him.

During colonial times, the public-school-educated British

judges would have had none of this nonsense. In a self-defence case, the actions of the accused were normally assessed by an objective standard – would the accused fear imminent physical harm if he was a 'reasonable, ordinary' man on what the judges called 'the Clapham Omnibus'. I doubted that most of the judges who wrote this had ever been on an omnibus, but they made it quite clear that this imaginary individual was on a bus being driven down a street in *England*, where nobody believed in ridiculous things like voodoo – rather than a dusty road in some faraway corner of the Empire.

Emerging from the colonial era, courts began to take a different view. 'The purpose of the criminal law is to punish an individual for his wrongdoing and not to sacrifice a few in the hope of converting their community from beliefs, however primitive, which they hold so deeply,' wrote a Ugandan judge in 1975. 'Criminal responsibility has always been individual.' The suspect could, he opined, claim self-defence, based on a reasonable belief that he was being attacked by voodoo. Another Ugandan case took a different approach, ruling that such a belief could provide a defence of insanity, as the belief was totally irrational.

I would side with the second judge: Willie certainly believed he was threatened by a hex, but to accept that as self-defence would mean it was real and would encourage others to respond to their fears in a similarly violent way. What we are trying to achieve in the law is to prompt non-violent responses to our fears, whether they are rational or irrational. If Willie had gone to a therapist rather than for a gun, the two victims would be alive today.

Meanwhile, Dad's latest booklet suggested that he was moving towards a genuine belief that reincarnation was a fact. I thought this was nonsense, yet people should be free to think what they like – the Archbishop of Canterbury may commune with his imaginary friend – so long as they do no harm. The same principles apply to Karl Marx, but we must draw a line when someone asserts the right to kill the capitalists with whom we disagree. Such a belief is deranged.

The law finds it hard to grapple with this, largely because the law wants to be violent itself – and impose harsh punishments. In 1901, the case of Solomon Notema came before the US Supreme Court. He had read his Bible, Leviticus 20:27: 'A man also or woman that hath a familiar spirit, or that is a wizard, shall surely be put to death: they shall stone them with stones.' The mandate from God could hardly be clearer: a local woman insisted she was a witch, so Notema killed her. The trial judge charged the jury that if Notema's belief both in witches and in his right to kill them was the product of a diseased brain – an insane delusion – he was not responsible and was entitled to an acquittal by reason of insanity. If, on the other hand, his belief was simply an erroneous conclusion of a sane mind, he was responsible and should be found guilty. He was found guilty as charged.

Notema (and Willie) genuinely believed something that was mad. He needed treatment, because we must make sure that kind of thing does not happen.

In the end, Willie's case turned on another form of madness: the same kind of racism that I had encountered at the Klan rally in Mississippi some years before. There is a tendency to say that racists are just bad – as many said my father was bad – but to designate yourself as superior just because your skin is white is just an example of a deranged mind, conceptually quite close to thinking you are God.

In an American trial, there is a 'voir dire' process when the lawyers get to question each juror about attitudes that may be relevant to the case, as part of the process ending with the twelve who will hear the case. Typically, there is an instruction given to members of the panel by the judge that reads: 'Voir dire is an ancient Latin phrase that means to speak the truth.' It is Old French rather than Latin, and it is better translated as 'to see, to say', which reflects its true nature. You listen to what they say, and watch their responses; you get to know them. And would we not all rather be judged by someone we know than a random stranger who might have any number of unknowable prejudices?

I love this part of the trial: you get to talk to people about their true beliefs, which allows you both to understand them and to learn to speak to them in a language that they may understand. Anyone can be excluded for 'cause' for an outright bias: for example, if the juror already thinks that the person on trial is guilty. On top of this, both sides get a certain number of 'peremptory' challenges where they can remove jurors for any reason or no reason. It was this type of challenge that caused problems. White prosecutors would get rid of as many black jurors as possible, so that the black person on trial would sit with his white court-appointed lawyer, staring disconsolately at the white judge and the jury of twelve people who would judge him, all of them white.

Willie Gamble's trial began two weeks after the Supreme Court decided *Batson* v. *Kentucky*, holding – finally – that something meaningful had to be done about prosecutors' racism. Under the new rule, the prosecutor had to give reasons for striking black jurors. The response by the two prosecutors in Willie's case was both unsurprising and shocking. Over a few drinks at a local cocktail party, one of the prosecutors explained what he had done to another lawyer, who later reported it back to me. 'The Supreme Court in Wash-ing-turn may say what they wur-nt,' he said, the words slurred in part by the accent, in part by the mint julep, 'but ah tha-nk it's . . . uh . . . un-con-sti-tu-shun-all to tell us how we kin use our challenges. We thawt we'd make this a test case.'

This attitude illustrated how long it sometimes takes for the real world to filter down to rural Georgia. The Supreme Court had said it, so it was by definition constitutional. When we picked Willie's jury, there were ten black jurors and the prosecution had ten peremptory strikes; they used their ten strikes on the ten black people. In one of the rare occasions when my endless years of maths was of use, I whipped out my calculator and – instructing a rather bewildered Judge McMillan on the finer points of Sir Ronald Fisher's hypergeometric distribution – pronounced the statistical probability of this pattern at roughly 6.7×10^{-20} or 0.000000000000000000067. In other words, they were being racist.

McMillan had been elected district attorney for six years himself, before being voted in as a judge, but he knew that he now had to demand that his old friends give their reasons for each strike. The first person they had eliminated from the jury was a Mr Mosely, who was struck, the prosecutor said, because he was a Mason, and there might be an issue in the case concerning Masonic Lodge affiliation. 'The prosecutor's explanation that Juror Mosely is a Mason is unpersuasive,' the Supreme Court of Georgia later admonished. 'Another black juror apparently was struck because he was a *brick* mason.'

The next black juror was – wait for it – Isaiah Mason. Their stated reason, they said, was that they could get no information out of him during their voir dire questioning: the Supreme Court pointed out that this was unsurprising, since they 'asked *no* questions of him'.

When it came to Juror Davis, one of the prosecutors said: 'I saw him pull into a known drug distribution centre, stay there briefly, then leave.' When pressed to identify this notorious spot, he admitted that the prospective juror had been filling up his vehicle at the Dixie gas station. I went to talk to the owner, a white man who became increasingly choleric as I described what the DA had been saying about his place of business. He came to the courthouse threatening a defamation writ.

And so it went on, down the entire list. Indeed, it seemed as if the prosecutors were taking the mickey – creating the most extreme example of racial bias they could. Predictably, their old friend Judge McMillan refused to find that they were being racist and let the trial move forward. However, their effort was so embarrassingly bad that even the Georgia Supreme Court (not known for its liberalism) reversed the conviction and Willie got a new trial, where we were able to work out a plea to something less than death.

If Willie should be deemed 'mentally ill' for an interpretation of voodoo that led him to take two lives, how should the line be drawn, and enforced, if the prosecutors used their own racist beliefs (that black people should not be allowed to sit on a jury) to try to kill him? The prosecutors would certainly bridle at the suggestion that they were deranged, though that is not as outlandish as it might initially sound. As recently as 18 March 2019, the United States Supreme Court considered the Georgia capital case of Keith Tharpe. His wife, Migrisus, had left him. He was not happy. He seemed to share my father's views about women and their duty to their husbands, though he went further in enforcing them. As Migrisus and her sister, Jacqueline Freeman, drove to work, he pulled his truck in front of their car and forced them to stop. He aimed a shotgun and ordered his wife to get into his truck. He then took Freeman to the rear of his truck and shot her, rolling her body into a ditch.

One might well wonder whether – however tragic – the murder of someone in the throes of Tharpe's anger was really the kind of extraordinary case that should send someone to the death chamber. It was enough for a panel of Jones County jurors – in particular for one white man, Barney Gattie. He had not revealed his racism during the jury selection process, but in the US – unlike the UK – it is totally legal to talk to jurors about their service. He signed an affidavit for Tharpe's appellate lawyer describing his views.

'There are two types of black people,' he opined. 'One, there are "black folks" and two, there are "niggers".' According to Juror Gattie, Jacqueline Freeman qualified as 'black folks';

Tharpe did not. Gattie expounded some more: 'Some of the jurors voted for death because they felt Tharpe should be an example to other blacks who kill blacks, but that wasn't my reason. After studying the Bible, I have wondered if black people even have souls.'

I doubt whether anyone has anything that might sensibly be termed a 'soul'. Yet it is a different degree of irrationality to think a person with light skin has a soul, while a person with a different hue does not. To date, every court has rejected Tharpe's bid for a new trial. 'It is indisputable among reasonable jurists that Gattie's service on the jury did not prejudice Tharpe,' wrote the Federal Court of Appeals, without any sense of irony.

I wondered where everyone stood on the spectrum of lunacy. 'Lunacy' – being touched by the moon – is a word I like. It makes little sense to say that Juror Gattie's view that a black person has no soul is merely an 'erroneous view held by a sane person', any more than we should validate the prosecutors' racism as somehow 'rational but wrong'. Rather, perhaps we should just consider which attitudes we are willing to accept, as they are harmless, as contrasted to the steps we need to take once a bizarre view threatens true damage.

The relatively easy part of the debate involves putting the victim in the position they were in before it happened – and this is particularly simple when it is a matter of government-sanctioned misuse of power, as with prosecutors or jurors. Hence, we can reverse Willie Gamble's death sentence because of the prosecutors' racism, and Keith Tharpe's because of Juror Gattie, and everyone goes back to square one, as well, we hope, as learning a lesson. The discussion becomes more complex when we focus on what action might be taken where the harm cannot be redressed. Willie took the lives of two people, yet Dad thought that was relatively inconsequential, as in his eyes those victims were now happily reincarnated. The challenge is to come up with a proper response to that – albeit not one that involves killing Willie to prove that killing is wrong.

18

The Edward Earl Johnson Libel

Sticks and stones can hurt my bones – but names can do far more damage.

Larry Lonchar had been convicted, rightly or wrongly, of murdering three people and trying to kill a fourth. However, harm to others comes in various forms. When it came to Dad, his venomous letters caused immense damage to those around him, and to his relationship with the world. If I were a gambler like Larry or Dad, I would bet that I will be condemned by some people who read that I once lost it with Cristiana, as I condemn myself, even if she said she did not even remember it the next day. Yet my words have caused much more damage to those about whom I care.

My 'Edward Earl Johnson libel' was perhaps the most damaging thing I have ever said, at least for Dad. The American notion of free speech is delimited by a simple rule: anything goes unless it is intended to provoke immediate physical violence. Maybe we should consider emotional violence too.

Merrilyn Thomas, a journalist with a local newspaper in Cambridge, had been captivated by the story of Edward Johnson's execution, and wanted to write a book about it. I had mixed feelings about the project: I would have liked to write such a book myself, as I owed it to Edward, but for now I did not have the time. After the documentary *Fourteen Days in May*, Paul Hamann did a follow-up called *The Journey* where he wired me up to talk to a man hanging out in a seedy Alabama motel who had likely pulled the trigger. A young woman told us that she was with Edward at the time of the murder: she had gone to the police, and had been told to buzz off and mind her own business. Naturally, she was black.

At the time, I subscribed to Mother Jones's motto – 'Pray for the dead and fight like hell for the living'. Since I could not do the job, I cooperated as best I could with Merrilyn in the hope that her investigative skills would uncover new evidence. I was sceptical, as I had driven her to Mississippi with her husband, David, and there had been a rare snowfall on icy roads; Merrilyn was spooked by this and, sitting in the passenger seat next to me, kept trying to pull the wheel in the wrong direction when I was trying to avoid skidding. We ended up in the ditch one time, though we got out without any harm done. But it seemed unlikely that she would confront some of Mississippi's angry law enforcement officers with the accusation that they had framed a black man for the murder of a white policeman.

Indeed, her book began to take a well-meant but unfortunate turn towards being as much about me, the Cambridge lad, as an exploration of what had led Edward to the gas chamber. She wrote to Dad for his views, without realising that he could be more of a challenge than any deputy sheriff. While we had driven around Mississippi, I had described the various things I have learned from him, albeit with a few health warnings.

'You refer to Clive as my "remarkable son",' Dad's reply began, 'and all I can reply to that is "heaven help the rest of humanity if you are right". If evolutionary development is to make real progress then each succeeding generation must achieve more than the mean of its parents and although it is always difficult to assess one's own doings, and although Clive may well be a late developer, I cannot see him achieving as much at his present rate as either of his parents in real terms. Like so much of today's talent a very little achievement has been magnified out of all proportion by some skilful media handling. I have always thought that, with far better opportunities than I had, neither Mark nor Clive has achieved as much at thirty as I had.'

I was not yet thirty, which may have escaped Dad's attention. A foolish vanity was increasingly infiltrating what Dad was writing, and it was uncomfortable, even embarrassing, as it made him look so bad.

'The system of Creation works through reincarnation and karma,' he continued. 'That is a fact not an opinion – which is why I keep telling Clive as politely as I can that the death penalty is not important. The law does not encourage original thinking and this is shown by the shambles which he made over Earl Johnson. So my honest opinion is that he is wasting his talent and may well miss his real potential completely if he does not make fundamental changes in his aims and standards within the next few months.'

He meant to copy me in, as – I think – he saw all this as simple fact, stated in a rather witty way, rather than something that might give offence. However, I did not see his letter for some decades. Dad was still living in the flat in Marbella, short on pesetas, and had taken to reducing his expenses by sending letters to Mum with instructions to send copies to all. Mum did not complain at his peremptory demands, as it allowed her to act as intermediary – and as censor.

'I suppose I had better send you this letter Clive's father has written to you,' she wrote to Merrilyn, as she knew she had to pass it on – otherwise he would only get angry and spend more time on his next screed. 'It tells you more about him than about Clive! He is regrettably manic just at the moment, and until this phase passes I am afraid you won't get much sense from him. I shan't send a copy to Clive – that seems quite unnecessary.'

As often happened when Mum made a well-intentioned intervention, this left me confused when I got my next letter from Dad. 'I am afraid I am a little in the doghouse with Mum for explaining (under extreme pressure!) a few of the facts of life,' he said. I had no idea what he was talking about. I paid it little thought, as his missive veered onto a rather Freudian theme about how his mother, Trix, was an excellent lover – I wondered how he knew, and whether his gay father, Albert, would have agreed. 'This evening I have literally not even one peseta which tests my faith to the limit. I am still laughing!'

This is when I committed my own cardinal sin. I had no idea of the consequences of my action, but what I was about to do precipitated a year of misery for my entire extended family.

Merrilyn mentioned that Dad had made some pointed comments. I told her not to take them too seriously. She said how Mum had already explained that he was bipolar. I said that this was true. 'The great sadness about Dad, I suppose, is that he has all these ideas, but they never come to anything. I don't think there is a single plan that has come to fruition in his whole life.'

Here was I, Dad's youngest son, passing judgement on him, saying that he was an utter failure. In my defence, it did not occur to me that she would put anything of the sort in her book, as I had only been giving her background so she would not get too carried away by whatever she might have heard from him. Yet my defence does nothing to mitigate the hurt of such a statement. If Dad's depression was based in part on his deep insecurity, few verdicts could have been more damaging.

Merrilyn did not quote me verbatim, but her own judgement of Dad was only disguised by English euphemisms. On page 34 of her book there was a brief description of Dad as a man 'with an original mind, whose failing was that he never managed to live up to his own high standards'. Page 35 contained a single sentence of relevance: 'Dick Stafford Smith departed from Cheveley Park Stud and his family, leaving his wife and sister to try and salvage the business from financial ruin.'

I only skimmed through the book when it came out – I was

disappointed that it contained no new evidence in Edward Johnson's case.

I was the one who sent Dad a copy of the book, signed by Merrilyn, to the apartment in Marbella. I did not think twice about it. It arrived a couple of days before he was forced to leave Spain – deported in part because he had been violent to Dawn, his second ex-wife, and in part due to the harassing letters concerning his SAPPSA project that he fired at King Juan Carlos.

He read the book through, stewed, and then spent much of the night tearing into a letter to Merrilyn, entitled 'Truth and the Responsibility of Authorship'. At the top he put the time he began (1 a.m.): it was several pages, so his two-finger typing must have consumed most of the time until sunrise. It was in red, meaning that he was particularly impecunious and the black half of the ribbon had expired. When I held it up to the sun, the page was splattered with starlight where machine-gun bullet holes appeared from each letter 'o', thumped by his heavy fingers.

'Clive was kind enough to send me a copy of your book *Life on Death Row* and since it bears your inscription as well may I thank you for your share in the gift?' he began, the first sentence of a battle that would last for many months. 'I have just finished reading it so I am afraid that this is likely to be the limit of my thanks since I think that the publication of the book has probably done a considerable disservice to the professional careers of two members of my family, including that of its head.'

For now, I was assumed to be a victim rather than a perpetrator. 'If Clive intends becoming a chat-show entertainer then it will not do him much harm and in the ambience of the States it may even help him,' Dad went on. 'But if, as I hope, he wants to become a serious professional then I fear that the damage may be considerable. Anyone who reads your book will see that you have painted the boy as a cross between an untrained idiot, who goes on making the same mistake time after time, and a sentimental teenager. However hard I stretch my paternal imagination, it is impossible to claim that he is very bright, but it was a little unkind of you to have advertised the fact in such a public manner. I love Clive very sincerely and I hate to see his future treated in such a cavalier manner.'

He continued detailing how I was to blame for Edward Johnson's death. I was equally guilty of killing Leo Edwards, who had been executed the following year – perhaps more so, since I was such a fool that I had not learned from my blatant mistakes.

Hitherto his letter had been a fusillade against Merrilyn dressed up as a fairly insulting pseudo-defence of me. He now turned to the two sentences which he would obsess over for months to come.

'May I also just mention the disservice you have done to me and to my professional and family situation?' Overnight, he had written up a revisionist version of the years 1965–79, exonerating himself entirely of any blame for the demise of the stud. 'The facts concerning the last days of my family at Cheveley Park Stud (which I still miss like a lost right arm) are not quite the same as you have stated. I could cheerfully wring your beautiful neck for having perpetrated such a stupid and ill-mannered libel.'

In red felt tip he scrawled at the end, 'I would suggest that you withdraw all books and remove the offensive pages, or insert a slip making a complete correction and apology.'

Until Mary pointed it out, I had missed the fact that Dad was now signing off all his letters – whether to me, Merrilyn or King Juan Carlos, no matter what the vitriol within – 'Have fun!'

When I first got my copy of Dad's letter, by fax, I groaned. It was soon followed by others demanding £1 million in damages and £25,000 for Mary for a 'slight by association'. To prevent

Merrilyn from being harassed by endless letters I hastened to send an ameliorative message. I had just seen Mary in Los Angeles and I assured Dad that her reputation, like mine, would be overvalued at twenty-five cents on the open market. I invited him over to the US as I thought that would divert him.

It did not have the desired effect. Dad was now lashing out. Auntie Jean made the mistake of debating with him. He obsessed over a single word in the book – that the stud had needed to be 'salvaged' – and they had a long telephone call. Dad insisted on his version of the truth. She recapped the long, sorry history of the stud's collapse, but went on to point out how not one of his subsequent ideas had got off the ground, essentially repeating what I had said.

When Dad called me I was too surprised to avoid him. I have a phobia of the phone. This was one of the rare occasions when Dad had enough coins to feed into the phone, and I remember the conversation well because, predictably, he imme-diately reduced his side of it to a letter.

'In the past month, you see,' he began, 'I've had letters from two friends of mine, though I've not yet met either. One is from your days at Columbia Law School, and the other more recently in the Supreme Court. They both believe that you are in danger . . . and I mean imminent danger . . . of bringing your profession into disrepute.'

'Yeah, Dad, right,' was all I said. I did not even ask him who these figments were. I knew it was total nonsense.

Dad's voice was jolly, the tone he had taken to using when he said something hurtful, as if he were making a light joke. 'Everyone was of one mind, you see – that you simply cannot be allowed to continue to disgrace both yourself and your pro-fession as well as your family in this way. If you recall I had told you that I could definitely have got both Edward Earl Johnson and Leo Edwards pardoned – and now I have this opinion from two of the most senior jurists that you should have done it within the rules of the law.'

I was not sure what to make of it all. It was sad. I wondered how he had convinced himself that such conversations had actually taken place – had he harangued someone in a pub, or was this just a musing from the bathtub? The rest of the call was devoted to the stud. I tuned out as it was all ancient history – though his version, while ancient, was not history. In the end, we talked briefly about him coming to Atlanta, and the call ended quietly. He knew I had not been agreeing with him, even though I had said little or nothing, so he immediately banged out a lengthy letter, again with bullet-hole 'o's all the way through, spattered with his inability to spell particular words: 'bankrupcy' and 'shitzophrenia'.

He added a postscript in red felt-tip which emphasised what the real issue was: 'Half the stud was to have been mine and I lost that! And I have also lost the comfort of my family, and it now appears their love and respect too.' He ended, 'Give my love to Cristiana and Have fun!' Cristiana and I had been apart for a long time by then.

I tossed the letter aside. I did not give it much thought. I should have – he was wreaking havoc in Newmarket, which had no impact on me since I was 4,000 miles away, but Mum was the primary victim.

As he had in 1963, Dad took to the media himself to repair the damage done by the 'libel' – by repeating it. The *Newmarket Journal* published an interview with him, shouting the headline 'FATHER AT WAR OVER SON'S BOOK!' It appeared on 12 October 1989, but I read it first twenty-eight years later, in 2017, when I came across it in my mother's papers – she had censored it for my sake. My first reaction was astonishment that any paper would publish such a thing without picking up the phone to check their facts with others involved.

'The book makes it seem that I deserted the ship and left huge debts. That wasn't the case at all,' Dad was quoted as saying. He announced that Merrilyn and I were defaming his good name, and that he was planning to join a 'gang of Ku Klux Klan Southerners' after my blood. He thought he would get me first. 'Clive's got to realise that, in some cases, the death penalty is essential,' he concluded.

Though Mum would normally hold back, knowing full well that a response would only provoke more misery, she accepted one of his calls. He was delighted that his interview had been featured so 'prominently'. She pointed out it was in a minor local publication, beside an advertisement for the West Suffolk Crematorium. Then she laid into him about some of the other things that might have been in the book, like the times he had beaten his mother, Dawn and herself. When he began to explain the 'extreme provocation' that led to his 'little slap', she hung up.

He called again, over and over, until she eventually decided to talk again. (She would almost always note down what they both said in the vain hope that reminding him later would somehow help her win an argument.)

'As far as you going on about how this book ruins your life in Spain is concerned,' she started, 'you've been deported, so you're mad if you think you currently have a future there.' The word 'mad' never went over well with Dad. His foot lunged onto the accelerator as he launched into a peroration about how everyone around him was ill.

'I accept that I am not normal,' he said. 'I mean, no one else works twenty-two hours a day. My God, woman, don't you see how warped you are . . . hell hath no fury! I mean, do you not see how I attempt to get those I love to behave properly . . . how I forgive them time and time again when they do not? I would not wish to be normal and nor would I wish my children to be normal if it can possibly be avoided in a world where the "normal" is so appallingly low.'

Mum was having none of this. 'Over the past seventeen years I know how fortunate I am that we parted. But here I am talking about the far more potent fury of a mother. Your denigration of them makes you a laughing stock, particularly when you suggest that you could make a better job of the work they are doing – it is absolutely ludicrous!' She had rummaged in her filing cabinet and promised to send him the mental health reports on him that she had stored over the years. She told him that if he continued his attacks, she would send copies of these to the *Newmarket Journal* in defence of her children.

Dad was, of course, feeling totally lost. The more he tried to get everyone to see the world his way, the more he drove them away. Mum would argue with him, which was at least interaction. I just found it tedious and refused to engage, which was worse.

At Christmas, I flew home to see the family. Dad had only lasted a few days in Newmarket, where he would always impose himself on Michael Fields, a jockey-sized friend from his schooldays. Michael would rarely complain, but we would try to get Dad somewhere else before their friendship was permanently dissolved. The small Cambridge flat Mary and Mum had lined up for Dad was on a large traffic island encircled by the Milton and Chesterton roads, across from the Victoria Avenue bridge. The flat had recently been painted white, but it was rapidly becoming less habitable as Dad kept burning toast and cooking kippers. The city was gloomy too, with English rain seeping into the pores. I took him some provisions, sent by Mum, and sat down for a cup of tea. He was still banging on about the 'libel'.

'Are you willing to give me a written statement?' he demanded, leaning forward in that intense way he had; his white hair was almost as wild as Einstein's. 'I have asked for it time and time again, to clear me of this calumny about the stud.'

He was sitting in one of the two armchairs, which was draped with an old green velvet tasselled covering that I recognised from my bed at Cheveley Park Stud, many years before.

Most of the other furnishings were also familiar, well-worn items on loan from Mum when he moved in.

I tried to change the subject, but he would not be diverted. In the end, I was faced with no exit – either I had to agree that Mum and Auntie Jean were the evil players in the tableau, which I could not possibly do, or I had to explain why not.

'Dad, I agree that it was stupid to put those things in the book,' I said. 'I agree that it added nothing. The problem is I was there, and you were the cause of the stud going bankrupt.' I waited for the explosion, but it did not come. He seemed stunned into silence. So I went on. 'All those bank loans. I remember very vividly a letter I wrote to you when I was thirteen, when you wanted to borrow more money. None of us wanted you to do it. Mark was against it, and I remember doing some fairly childish maths on it myself – how much would be owed on the interest alone before anyone even began to pay back the bank. It was impossible, it wasn't going to work out, and the oil crisis didn't help – nobody but the Arabs were able to dabble in thoroughbreds. It's not just me who thinks that, or Mark and Mary, it's everyone. As far as we are all concerned, it is just a fact. An old fact, which does not matter any more.'

I continued, trying to soften the blow. I was very glad, I said – and meant it – that the stud had gone bankrupt. My life would have been very different had this not been the case. I gained two things: first, the knowledge that our new-found family wealth, inherited from Robert Sherwood, had brought no happiness; and second, the certainty that I wanted nothing to do with riches myself. Nobody was now blaming him for anything; we were all getting on with lives that were much happier.

We finished our tea. It seemed to work. However, just as Dad had his fantasy world, the idea that telling the truth would achieve my goal was my delusion. He called Mum and spoke of the delightful time he and I had enjoyed. I met with him every day I was home, and he oscillated. On the third visit to a pub, he agreed it was all ancient history and we should drop it. The next time I saw him, the drumbeat of libel was back.

Back in Atlanta there was a strange spate of bomb scares – a white supremacist was threatening to kill lawyers who dared represent black men accused of raping white women. It was tedious. I returned to my house to find a bulge under the door-mat, a cubical package with a return address in New Jersey. I decided that if it had been delivered through the post it should not detonate easily before being opened, so I shook it gently, provoking a metallic jangle. I put it back down and went to track down the company on the return label.

Had they had sent me a package? No. Oh dear, this height-ened my concern.

Before calling in the ATF – the federal Bureau of Alcohol, Tobacco and Firearms – I thought I had better probe some more, so I asked them to check anything to my postal code.

Yes, there was one from a Samuel Johnson, they said. What was the return address? 'Parchman, Mississippi.' Death row. At that point, I dared to open it. Sam had very thoughtfully and at considerable expense sent me a pair of Chinese Baoding balls, designed to reduce tension. Sam happened to call the next day, and I told him that my stress level had been raised several points by the experience.

Dad's obsession with the 'libel' gradually faded into the back-ground. One day, his habit of hand-delivering 'important' letters took him out first-thing to Cherry Hinton, on the out-skirts of Cambridge.

'I have just got back from a most enjoyable walk in a day which turned out to be fairer than the forecast suggested it would be,' he wrote to his sister Jean. He described walking by the asylum at Fulbourn, where he had mulled over the various opinions that had been expressed about his lifetime of failure. 'After what has happened to me, I feel very much in sympathy with the poor dear, our grandmother. The "attack" over the past months has been difficult. It is sad to find the children converted to the opposition but do not think that state will last long. I feel I am the only person to bring a sense of reality and common sense into a situation of cloud cuckoo land, and yet various people see me as being in need of rapid psychiatric help. The trouble is, whose sense is sense, and whose logic is logical?'

19

The Samaritans: What Is Our Duty to People Who Want to Take Their Own Life?

O the mind, mind has mountains; cliffs of fall
Frightful, sheer, no-man-fathomed. Hold them cheap
May who ne'er hung there.

Gerard Manley Hopkins, 'No worst, there is none'

It was Good Friday. It meant only hot-cross buns to me, but to Dad it was a potent day in the calendar.

'A sadly appropriate day on which to write this letter,' he wrote to his sister:

You have, I am afraid, always had to pick up the pieces of your brother's irratic [*sic*] and illogical behaviour and try to explain to yourself and to others. I am sorry to have to ask you to do it again. I have decided overnight there is really no future in going on in the muddle of my life. Self-justification has always been my forte. I have done unnecessary harm to those around me – not least to you and to the children. As far as I am capable of love I have loved you all but I believe looking back that somewhere along the line I lost the ability of genuine love. I am basically such an inadequate little brat that I have never learned to love myself and therefore never got beyond first base. I am sure that SAPPSA – like all the other projects I thought would long ago justify myself in my own eyes, and rehabilitate my tarnished reputation in the eyes of those with whom I have lived – is not going to come through. I am now so mentally sick that I know that I am not going to be able to pick up the pieces and start again.

This is the only letter I shall leave. Can you do what you can to explain what I am doing so that it causes the least long-term damage to the children? Maybe there is a genetic flaw somewhere in the family in which case they are probably best to face up to it openly with the help of modern medicine and not try to brush it under the carpet as I did when the university tried to intervene all those years ago. On the other hand my problems may have been started by the car accident and aggravated by another knock I got on the head in South Africa during the war. Or both these may be just another self-justification to cover a weak and useless character – I don't know but I may do in a few hours when all is hopefully revealed.

I move on still believing in reincarnation and an existence after death. So hope springs eternal even if it is now based on another plane of existence.

For perhaps the first time in a few years, Dad did not sign off about having fun: 'I leave you all my love – such as it is. Dick.'

When Jean received this, she was desperately worried. Nobody had phoned. Perhaps he had gone somewhere in the woods, and his body would not be found for weeks? She made several calls, panicked.

She eventually tracked him down, to find he had fortunately failed in his plan to take his own life.

Earlier, when I was still a teenager, and we had moved to the little house on Clarendon Street in Cambridge, Mum would be gone at least one evening a week. She was volunteering with the Samaritans. She did not speak about it much, and never told stories about the people who called in. She did it because she understood. She had been there for Dad. Mark had sat on the bed when Dad described the black dog that haunted him; Mary had borne the brunt of it. I had sailed blithely through Dad's depressions, unaware. My only black dog had been Vesta, our Labrador.

With Larry Lonchar, though, I finally had to face up to what my duties were. He was on death row now, and had been forced by law to suffer through a pointless appeal to the Georgia Supreme Court. William Warner, then his lawyer, came to me asking if I could take over the case. I have never been good at saying no – I said I would do the next stage to the US Supreme Court. There was, Bill warned, a roadblock in the way: Larry would not consent to filing any appeals, as he wanted to die and get it all over with. At the time, I was twenty-seven, and I knew everything there was to know. I rolled out the lecture I had once heard from Millard Farmer.

'Don't worry about it, Bill,' I airily pronounced, swivelling my chair from side to side. 'Everyone says it sooner or later. We call it their New Hampshire licence-plate moment – "Live Free or Die".'

'I'm not sure this is the same thing,' Bill said tentatively, from the shabby green leather seat opposite me. 'He seems awful sure about it.' He was fifteen or more years my senior, the hair around his warm round face already touched by grey, as he reflected on the certainty of my youth. He was a little put off by the chaos in my office: the building cleaners never had to hoover the floor as they could not see it. But Bill had never before done a death penalty case, and non-capital lawyers tended to approach the small clique of capital defenders as if we were the Delphic Oracle, no matter how young we were.

'Don't worry,' I repeated. 'It's a cry for help. You want my theory on it?' I paused just long enough to be polite, though the unfortunate man had no chance to say no. 'Ego is built, in reality or in myth, on the notion that you make decisions, choices. You sit in your cell, and gradually you lose every choice you ever had. You don't get to "choose" when you get up, when you eat, when you shower, even when you take a crap, for Christ's sake. And as you lose your choices, your sense of self starts to ebb away.

'And it's all reinforced from the free world as well. You're on death row, nobody comes to see you, ever. Sometimes, for a long time, you don't even have a lawyer. And everyone keeps telling you how you're worthless. So finally you're left with only one choice that only you unquestionably can make. And that's when you choose to die.'

I paused again, this time for dramatic effect, sure that somewhere Sigmund Freud was nodding sagely. 'So you choose to die. That's all that gives meaning to your life. The choice between life and death. But the moment you make it, the papers have your name on the front page, all us do-gooder liberals come rushing down to stop you, and you suddenly discover that life has meaning for you after all. So you take your appeals back up. What we have to do is make sure that we have enough people there visiting, and keeping Larry cheerful, so he doesn't get back to his state of nihilism.'

Quod erat demonstrandum, I wanted to say; the elegant mathematical equation proved itself.

'Well, I hope you're right,' Bill said sceptically.

It was true that most of my clients wanted to drop their appeals at one point or another, and we were gradually developing ways to keep the clients on board with our legal strategies. Edward Johnson's execution had spawned an organisation called Lifelines, where several hundred folk had taken up writing to the people on death row. This meant that pen pals wrote every week to most of the prisoners, where often family members did not. My mother was writing to Tracy Hansen, one of my men on death row in Mississippi. This human interaction helped to keep people alive.

But Larry was different.

Soon after my conversation with Bill, I got to meet Larry Lonchar for the first time. I drove the forty miles down to the

Georgia Diagnostic and Classification Center. I got there before 8 a.m., with time for a cup of weak coffee in the diner at the gas station just off I-75. Light brown plastic bench seats framed the red Formica tables, with a view over the pumps. I often had a rendezvous there with other people who were visiting death row.

I got back into my car for the two hundred yards to the main gate. The guards waved me in, and I drove another four hundred yards with pine trees on my left, the massive walls of the prison behind metal fences on my right. There was an artificial lake, draining through to a smaller pond and then back to the original stream. The soil was poor, but trusted inmates in their blue-striped prison uniforms struggled among the sparse flowers. Only around the main tower did the impatiens grow with abandon.

I parked in the visitor lot, waved at the guard looking out of the tower window, and waited to be buzzed through the entrance gate. This led through one set of metal detectors, followed by fifty yards of neon lights in the yellow tunnel, to the stairway at the end that led up to the main level. I had stripped down to the bare essentials – even cheap shoes, and a plastic belt that would make it through the security without me having to take it off. Up two steps at a time, I arrived at the second security area, through another metal detector. Here, they stamped something on my wrist that would show up under the ultraviolet scanner when I left. This was intended to foil an escape if, as had once happened, a visitor swapped clothes with a prisoner. Once through, I chose a seat to the right of the double electric gates that protected the visiting area from the depths behind. I knew that guards would eventually march Larry along the hallway from Cell Block G, ordering him to a halt beside the bulletproof glass of the control centre. From where he stood, Larry could survey the plastic seats beyond to see who was there.

It always took them forty-five minutes to amble a hundred

yards to fetch a prisoner. I used to memorise sonnets and extracts of Shakespeare and Dante to pass the time among the breeze blocks. Eventually, the yellow steel of the barred gate slid to the right. I watched Larry: I would come to know his trademark walk, swaying from side to side, kicking the flat soles of his tennis shoes up. He almost goose-stepped his way through the gate, as he gazed steadfastly at the ceiling. Eventually, he allowed them to sheepdog him into the long visitation room. He politely said hello.

I explained who I was, and he indicated that he already knew: the pond of capital defence is a small one. 'Yeah. Seen you down here visiting . . . Brandon. That's right. Brandon Jones.' Brandon was in a cell a few down from Larry. 'Don't know what they sent you here for,' he said lugubriously, but without offence. 'I ain't gonna let nobody file no appeal. You gotta know that.'

I said Bill Warner had asked me to take on his case.

'Bill Warner, now he's a good man. I like him,' Larry said. 'But Bill must've told you, I ain't taking no more appeals.'

I had not planned to talk about appeals for an hour or two. Maybe not even at all that day, if that's what it took. I had brought the necessary documents for Larry to sign, concealed among some poems in a manila file, just in case he caved in faster than expected. It would spare me another trip. But I had budgeted this to be just a social visit. Few people surrendered at once, as that would mean a loss of face. It would take a little trust.

We talked about sports. Larry loved University of North Carolina basketball, even if their football team had let him down on his bets. I boasted about hurling a snowball at Mike O'Koren, one of UNC's illustrious basketball alumni, a seven-foot giant who had chased after me. I did not want to push my luck. I read the American sports pages mainly to be able to hold up my end of a conversation in jail. Larry quickly placed me as a fake fan.

Larry was equally happy bemoaning the state of American politics. A surprising proportion of my white clients were knee-jerk Republicans, an inheritance that never got erased by Ronald Reagan's calls for faster executions. It was a relief to find, in Larry, a northerner who understood unions and the plight of the blue-collar worker.

I left without even bringing up the subject of his appeal. That was not what he expected. The second time I went to see him, he almost signed on just because I never asked him to – I judged the time not ripe. Larry appreciated a good game of poker, but he decided not to fold that easily.

We had ninety days to file the appeal, and the third time I visited him they were almost up. I brought the petition with me. It looked impressive – twenty pages of legal argument, neatly formatted. I was laying down what looked like a full house. It was a prefabricated one. Thanks to the new computer system, it had probably taken me only six hours to complete. I had not even begun to review Larry's case properly. I knew from the direct appeal that he had a good chance of a new trial, but I had no idea whether he might one day see freedom.

'Larry, c'mon! I've already done all the work. Won't you let me file the damn thing?' I tried not to whine. I had Larry pegged as a decent guy who would not want to make me waste my time. For an hour, he wavered. His arguments were quite basic. He did not want to spend life in a Southern prison. He harboured a simmering distaste for the Southern prison guard, whom he would have described as having shit–kicker cowboy boots; faded, oil–stained blue jeans; and the redneck's large, round stomach, lined with pork bellies and grits, hanging over an engraved leather belt. In Larry's mind, the buckle probably read 'SON-o-the-SOUTH' entwined around a Confederate flag. The greasy uncombed hair would be partially obscured by a cap with a high-water mark from the sweat stains. More likely than not, the brown filth of the tobacco plug would be wedged in between stained molars and his bulging cheek, and he would spit next to your ankle – Larry despised chewing tobacco. Above all else, Larry's stereotypical obese Southern guard ran a prison full of snitches. Unlike in Michigan prisons, where snitches had to be confined to the protective custody cells for their own safety, in a Georgia cell block it was impossible to organise prisoner solidarity.

'What do they think they're gonna get by doin' what they're told? These people're trying to kill us!' Larry's voice rose to a high note on the word 'kill' as he dared say what so many pretended to ignore. If people with similar interests could not stick together, then they were all *snitches*.

'Man, they're just a bunch of *inmates*. Not a *convict* among them.' Larry set much stock in his status as a convict, and spat the word 'inmate'. The actions of an *inmate* were designed to please his overseers – who were, Larry said, running a 'slave plantation'. Not so the convict. Respect power if he must, the convict would never cower to it. *Inmates* inhabited prisons; *convicts* ran them. A prison full of convicts would be a prison where gambling debts were paid. In contrast, an *inmate* in debt would put in for a transfer to another cell block, the institutional equivalent of declaring bankruptcy. *Inmates* were always running to teacher.

Whatever its morality, honesty was good policy with Larry. His antennae were always on alert for deception. Life in prison *was* an intolerable option, but it might be the only one available. So what should I say . . . what *must* I say to bring him to that point of view? Here – for the first time of many – I found myself in a moral quandary with Larry. Before me was a human being whom I immediately and instinctively liked, who was trying to kill himself. How far could I go . . . how far *must* I go to prevent him? What was my obligation to someone who wanted to kill himself – particularly someone who wanted to die the most torturous death imaginable, in the chair?

I beat a tactical retreat, and explained that even if we could not get him out (and I hoped we could), he could be sent to serve his sentence up north. The idea came to me in the middle of our conversation, but it might have been true. Once the show trial was over, Georgia had no real interest in paying to keep Larry. If Michigan was willing to take him, Georgia would gladly ship him home.

Larry wavered. His mother was now in Georgia, along with his brothers, Chooch and Tiny. His sister had moved to Florida. His father was the only one left in Michigan, and the chances of a visit from Milan Jr were no greater than the Grand Trunk Drunk Line running sober. I pointed out to him that he had never had visits from anyone at all when he was in prison there before.

He retired to the next line of defence. He did not want to spend life in *any* prison. There are two distinct halves to any capital case in the US – the culpability phase (did you do it?) and the punishment phase (you have now been shown to be guilty, so what is the punishment to be, life or death?). I pointed out to him that the issue I had included in his petition to the Supreme Court only challenged his conviction, not his death sentence. The Georgia court had clearly been wrong when it ruled he could be tried *in absentia*. So that meant if we won he would have a full retrial, and a chance of walking free. I promised him that if it came to that, I would do his retrial, rather than leave him in the hands of some public defender. In DeKalb County, in front of Judge Castellani, we would have a real chance.

Larry wavered some more. He told me that he had announced to the other men on death row that he was going out. I pretended that this was not significant, but inwardly I choked. He was painting himself into a corner. The convict's fear that he would lose face might march beside him into the death chamber.

Finally, he said he'd take the work I had done back to his cell and think about it. That was not good enough, as it was already due, but I could see I was not going to get any further, so I stopped badgering him, and we parted as friends.

I was annoyed as I drove the forty miles back to my office. As much as I was concerned for Larry, I was frustrated. Normally, I wrote a petition and the client signed off on it gratefully. Here was I, the busy lawyer, who had made *three* visits, and still he had not signed. Listening to my favourite Atlanta station, 96 Rock, I began to calm down. I preached patience to myself. If I could not go every week, I knew someone who could. I called Laura Patton, a law student who had been volunteering on Larry's case, and she agreed to visit him continually until he changed his mind.

Sure enough, ten days later I received the petition in the mail, along with the signed affidavit. 'I decided to go with it,' Larry wrote. 'You put a lot of work into this.'

That was so Larry. He hated to offend.

I was now his lawyer, and he allowed an appeal. I sent it to the Supreme Court, hoping they would not notice that it was two weeks late. Somehow, they never did. Neither did the 'Death Squad' in the Attorney General's office, the first of many occasions when they unwittingly helped to keep Larry alive. We had slipped under the radar. Larry was safe for the rest of the year. When the state finally got around to responding, I put a lot of work into the reply brief. I wanted to impress on Larry that he now had a team working for him.

The odds of getting the Supreme Court to take a case, while better than many bets Larry had taken, are always slim – perhaps 2 per cent.

Larry lost. The Supreme Court ruled in one word: *Denied*. Once again he plumbed the depths of his depression. Nine people up in Washington had decided his life was not worth saving.

The next step was generally an execution date. For no good reason, weeks and then months went by. Again, the very people who said they wanted to kill Larry seemed unwilling to make it happen.

20

Did Larry Even Do It?

Over time, naturally, you lose your innocence from gaining knowledge.

Albert Hammond Jr

At trial, Larry's lawyer, Cal Leipold, had battled as best he could with a recalcitrant client. He tried to raise questions about the third man. Nobody alive had actually seen what took place in the front room of the Smith condominium, and the puzzle that the prosecution sought to piece together had only two actors – Larry Lonchar and Mitch Wells. Various hints had come out at trial, though, that cast doubt on the prosecution's case. Amber Watson was Larry's probation officer. Even though she was horrified by the crime, it was difficult for her to believe the self-deprecating man she supervised had committed so cold an act. 'Larry said even the first news reports told how three people were seen leaving the scene,' she wrote in her report. Mitch Wells was one of the three. While Larry resignedly insisted he had been there, one plus one still only made two.

'Larry's mother had told me that Larry blamed his brother Paul for what had happened,' Amber Watson wrote in a second report. 'So I asked Larry why he blamed Paul. Larry said it was a long story, and would not say any more about that.'

It was well past time that I did some investigation into the case. I was going through the trial and appellate lawyers' cardboard boxes when I came across a discussion that Cal Leipold had at the jail with Larry, just two weeks before they were to pick the jury. Leipold had recorded the entire interview. Larry had been quite open.

There was a local man called Crumbley, a drug dealer, who owned the Desperado Bar. Larry thought – though he could not prove – that Crumbley had paid Mitch Wells and another person to kill Wayne Smith over some territory dispute. Larry had no weapons himself, he said. 'Wells had . . . he kept the guns . . . him and Dougie had three guns. One was . . . I know one was a big .357 or a .45. I'm not sure. I've known Dougie . . . he's my cousin. He's used to pulling bank jobs. One stays in the car and one pulls the robbery. So that's the thing.'

Mitch Wells had bought some handcuffs at the Army Surplus Store in Forest Park.

'Let me tell you something right off the bat,' Leipold said. 'Let me tell you something that's interesting. You know the knife that killed the woman? Somebody else's blood is on that knife.'

'Yeah,' Larry replied, non-committal.

'Well, you don't know that until now . . . I'm telling you that right now. Somebody else's blood is on the knife. You know whose blood it's not?'

'Yeah.' More emphatic this time. 'I know it's not mine.'

'It's not yours.' This stirred Larry from his torpor for a moment. The person who had cut up Margaret Sweat had left his own blood on the knife.

'The blood that's not hers?' Leipold asked. 'You know who else's blood it's not? It's—'

'Yeah.' Larry knew. It belonged to the person who had stabbed her.

'The blood type is wrong . . . It's not hers and it's not yours,' Leipold repeated. 'The question is, whose blood is it?'

Larry knew. But he was not naming names. Leipold should have held this conversation many months earlier if he was going to work Larry around to a name.

'How can I prove anything?' Larry moaned. 'I was sat right

next to that man Wayne – one foot – sitting right there on the couch, when he was shot.'

'Did they have guns in their hands when they—'

'Not when they first came in, no. Wells handcuffed Wayne.' Larry stopped. He had started talking, and was going further than he had intended to. 'Why are we going through this?'

'Because already you have given me at least four or five things that have helped me.' Leipold was not going to be put off. 'Wells handcuffs Wayne. What does the other guy do while Wells is handcuffing Wayne?'

'He's got him covered with a gun.'

'O K. Is anybody else handcuffed at that time?'

'Yeah.'

'Wells handcuffs Steve?'

'Yeah.'

'And then what happened?'

'Steve is standing above the chair, you know, Wayne – Wayne is still sitting down . . .'

'What's the woman doing?' Leipold wanted to understand what had happened to Margaret Sweat, as her stabbing – and the recorded emergency call – was probably the most difficult evidence that the defence faced.

'She went in the bedroom.'

'She went in the bedroom. Did they tell her to go in the bedroom?'

'Yeah.'

'They didn't handcuff her?'

'No. They only had two pairs of cuffs.'

'Then what happened?'

'. . . He shot Steve.'

'How many times?'

'I just seen him shoot once.'

'Where was Steve hit – could you tell?'

'Had to be in the front.'

'Chest, stomach, could you tell?'

'No.' It was hardly likely that Larry would have been spotting precisely where a bullet had passed, if all of this came as a total surprise.

'What next? Did Steve fall down when he was—'

'Yeah. Fell over the chair.'

'What about Wayne?'

'He turned, pointed – the other guy – I thought he pointed the gun at me,' Larry said. He and Wayne were only a foot apart. 'I . . . you know . . . froze, closed my eyes. I thought I was dead.'

'What about the other bedroom, not the bedroom the woman went to?' That would be where Charles was.

'Yeah,' Larry said. 'I heard two gunshots back there.'

'That's when Wells shot the kid who lived,' Leipold surmised. 'What happened next?'

'This other guy said, get Larry's billfold. Took my billfold, he took my keys, he took my glasses. I stood up and gave it to them. Wells went over to him, the couch right where Wayne died. It's not five feet from the door. It's right close to the door. So I stood up and gave it to him. You know, Wells and this guy . . . discussion. I – I just ran out the door. They chased me.'

'Who chased you?'

'Both of them.'

'Where did you go?'

'Towards the woods. I'm telling you, man, they tried to kill me. They took my glasses. They took my billfold. They took my money. Only way I got out of that house alive is . . . I thought they were going to kill me . . . I ran.'

If this was the case, Margaret would have been shouting to Larry – thinking he was outside and could save her, when actually he had made a run for it.

There was still the matter of the motive. The prosecution thought Larry was behind it all because he had to neutralise his $10,000 debt. Larry insisted that he was a convict, not an inmate, and he paid his bills. He was going to pay this one too.

'That morning . . . I was there . . . I took them $2,500,' Larry said. 'Was that found in the house?'

'Just stop a minute. Tell me what you're talking about.' Leipold prevented Larry from rambling on somewhere else. 'You took them a . . . an envelope with $2,500 in cash earlier that day, before everything else went down?'

'Yes.'

'For what purpose?'

'To help pay off the money I owed, and—'

'You took that with you that day?'

'Yeah. In the house. Not Wayne . . . but Steve,' he said. It had been earlier the same day. Wayne had not been there when he paid it. 'Like I said, Wayne's money – hell . . .'

'What kind of envelope was it?'

'Manila envelope.'

'Manila?'

'Yeah.'

Leipold was interested in how he got that kind of money. Larry explained he had seen no way to pay back Wayne Smith without getting into a bit of drug selling, in between his parole appointments.

'What are you saying, you sold eight ounces of cocaine?'

'See, I don't know nothing about drugs,' Larry said. 'Me and my brother went up to Battle Creek. You know, my brother is a heavy user of drugs.'

'That's Paul?'

Larry paused. He did not like to bring family into this.

'Yeah,' he said eventually. 'And we went up there . . .'

'When before the killing?'

'Few days . . . a week.'

'What are you telling me now? Are you telling me you want to take a polygraph test? I mean, let's not have me try to arrange this thing and get this guy over here and then have it fall through.'

'Like I say—'

'Do you want to do it?'

'Hey, I'll do one,' Larry said firmly, but rather disinterested. I was curious about that. Larry would not agree to something like a lie detector unless he was telling the truth.

Leipold had got a lot of useful material out of his client, if rather late in the day. He was annoyed that Larry had been speaking to other people too, including Amber Watson.

Larry began to talk about the days leading up to the crime. 'Amber remembered that I had an appointment . . . that she arranged an appointment. I was – this thing happened on Monday. I had an appointment with the psychiatric hospital for Wednesday, which she arranged. I wanted to die out there long before I wanted to die in here. I even told her. That's why she arranged this appointment.' It was not surprising that he had been so depressed – $10,000 in debt to Wayne Smith on top of everything else.

There was silence as Leipold digested this.

'I have no reason to be alive. She brought it up again just last night, why do you want to die? Well, I didn't want to live out there, did I? Because . . .' Larry's voice petered out. He didn't really want to talk about it.

'Larry, from the beginning when I talked to you, you have, as you know, repeatedly told me you want to die.'

'Yes.'

'You told a number of people you wanted to die.'

'Yeah.'

'What do you mean when you say that? Why do you want to die if you didn't do this thing?'

'Hey, I have my reasons,' Larry said. 'Like I say, this is – well, like I said, I can't gain nothing now, can't get Wells to admit it, my witnesses are dead. Like I say, my only defence – I can tell you right now, we can go to Battle Creek, the week before this I had eight ounces of cocaine. We can go – like I say, I can get witnesses, proof I had this dope deal set up. That blows everything. I had no reason for – for me to kill them people. We just arranged how we was going to Reno. But the only way I can prove anything is have Wells admit it. He's not going to get on the stand and admit he's been lying.'

Wells's version of events was basically the story the prosecution went with, though he radically limited his own culpability. According to him, Larry was the bad guy in all this, murdering three people to avoid his gambling debt.

'The only way, like I say, is trick him and have somebody be wired or the place we're at wired when we talk, you know,' Larry went on. 'If I can't prove nothing, I'm not – No. I'm gonna protect my family . . . 'cause I know those people will kill.'

'On the trial of your case, how do you feel about taking the witness stand, about testifying?' Leipold clearly thought, at last, that there might be some kind of a defence.

'What good if . . . I can't back nothing up?' Larry said. He had talked much more than he ever intended, and he was about to go back into his cave. 'I'm tired of people lying. I'm tired of – why do they want to fabricate shit like this? If they want to lie, hell, they can have my life. I don't care about my life, you know. I'm tired . . . I'm just tired. Hey, they – hey, they – hell, I should just plead guilty. They don't have to go through all that lying and shit. No wonder DeKalb County have that 97 per cent conviction rate if they gonna fabricate things.'

Looking back over this depressed me as well as giving me hope. There were inconsistencies, of course, as there are in everything – but the essence of what Larry said could very well be true; he might be innocent of the crimes. I already knew, from various things he had let slip, that he was covering for someone close to him – either because they were involved or because exposing the truth would bring the real killer down on his family. He had wanted to die before any of it happened, and maybe this was just a convenient way to make someone else do it for him. Could I ever move Larry towards the real hope that would keep him alive – first, that he could get out of prison, and second, even harder, make something of his life?

I needed to get out into the field, to do some investigation. Much as lawyers believe in their own silken tongues, my mistake in Edward Johnson's case had been to rely on legal technicalities. The facts are what rule any case. We had no money to hire an investigator, so I would be on my own. And I needed Larry's help, which was currently not forthcoming.

21

Colonel Humphrey Brooke and What It Means to Be Bipolar

[Manic depression] can only be cured by sex and smoking.
Lieutenant Colonel Humphrey Brooke

Auntie Jean had an unfortunate ability to say exactly the wrong thing to Dad at the wrong moment. It was understandable. I was across the Atlantic; she was constantly involved. She sent Dad an article from the *Observer* about manic depression (as bipolar disorder was then called), intending to push him to recognise his illness. It was titled 'Extremities of Mind: Humphrey Brooke describes the state of manic depression'. Once I identified the author, it became clear that Dad had found a soulmate.

Lieutenant Colonel Thomas Humphrey Brooke, CVO, was born in 1914, and was sent off to Wellington College, then to Magdalen College, Oxford, before he became a 'Monuments man' – as loosely portrayed in the 2014 George Clooney film. This was a dangerous yet glamorous moment at the end of the war when a British Special Operations Executive mission, code-named 'Bonzos', was tasked with saving the art that the Nazis had looted, some stored in Austrian salt mines. Hitler had issued his 'Nero Decree' – destroy it all so it does not fall into anyone else's hands – but the SOE assembled a local force, harassed the retreating Germans and helped to save various treasures.

Flowing from his experience, Brooke became deputy director of the Tate Gallery, as well as secretary of the Royal

Academy. However, in 1964, a bout of mania precipitated his early retirement. He took off to Suffolk, where he became an internationally acknowledged expert on roses. He grew over five hundred varieties, later opening his garden to the public, calling it 'the first rosarium in Great Britain'. His brief Wikipedia biography tells us that 'Brooke wrote an article for the *Observer* about his illness, which received over 150 responses'. Dad was one of those intrigued.

'Manic depressives tend to arouse strong feelings one way or another,' Brooke wrote in that article. 'We are opinionated, egotistical and verbose. We chain-smoke, which is socially unacceptable today. We make superhuman demands on our spouses, who need to be exceptionally intelligent and sympathetic. We send long, handwritten letters to all our friends.'

In addition to his entirely harmless obsession with roses and – from my perspective – an admirable love of cricket, he was consumed by an investigation into historical figures who may have suffered from manic depression. Generally, he insisted, the illness was rare and suffered almost exclusively by people of high education and intelligence. 'Everything that we call genius,' his psychiatrist told him, 'is manic depression in its non-depressive phase.'

Given that he was writing about himself, British modesty had to allow some room for lesser humans. 'Not all manic depressives are geniuses, but it is an illness which enhances even the most minuscule abilities.' In the non-depressive phase, the person's faculties – whether at bridge or poetry – are immensely enhanced.

He identified a number of musical geniuses – Schumann, Wagner, Mahler, Elgar, Rachmaninov – as manic-depressives, along with Winston Churchill, Edward Gibbon, Clive of India, Oliver Cromwell, William Wilberforce and Virginia Woolf. I had read a fair amount about manic depression because I always felt, looming in the background, the sword was hanging over my own head. When I found William Shakespeare in

Brooke's inventory, I began to suspect that his study had become inverted: not only were all manic-depressives brilliant, but if you were brilliant, you were, *ipso facto*, manic-depressive. His was a fantastically unscientific 'study' where nobody who was nobody could enter his pool.

Rightly enough, though, Brooke rued the fact that mania only needed an added 'c' to tar a bipolar person. Given that he had been ruled out of London life and dispatched to the country, Brooke searched for a cure. The *Sunday Times* suggested vitamin C, but he felt that was a placebo. He entered the ring for more than a hundred bouts with the electroconvulsive therapy machine, which he decided offered only a temporary lull. His psychiatrist had him take up to seventeen pills a day before Dr William Sargant gave him lithium, which he found stabilised him somewhat. However, most tellingly both for Brooke and my father, Gustav Mahler was supposedly roused from depression three times during his composition of his Third Symphony in 1896 by his sexual liaison with the beautiful soprano Anna von Mildenburg. In the end, then, Brooke came to the conclusion that his own manic depression 'can only be cured by sex and smoking'.

Some of what Brooke wrote made sense: some 'cures' offered by professionals seemed focused only on curtailing the patient, rather than seeking a way in which he or she could fit into the world with less friction on all sides. Yet if Brooke rued the word 'maniac', I rued his article. The notion that all genius was mania, and that the best response was more sex and smoking, was guaranteed to prevent Dad from any constructive approach to his situation.

I have, for twenty years, suffered from insomnia. I am wide awake at 4 a.m., never to return to slumber. I am paranoid about it and I have no qualms about medicating myself. Once, in a moment of insight, Dad told me I had to get my sleep. Perhaps he, like me, saw his depressive troughs partly as a natural end to a long high, when his body would insist on a rest. We can all operate on adrenaline for a while: I have had trials lasting three weeks where I would finish preparing at four in the morning and have to be up by seven. At the end, I crash.

Dad would not take his own advice, and preferred Brooke's. 'One of these rules of thumb is that we need eight hours' sleep a day,' he said to me on one occasion. 'But eight is for the average person. When I am operating efficiently, with a good sex life, I can go indefinitely on two hours. That is one hour at night and one at siesta – making love before and after on both occasions.'

Like Colonel Brooke, Dad was sure that frequent sex was integral to maximising the positive impact of his manic 'abnormality'. I was not the only recipient of his advice. He wrote to Baron Hemingford about one of his latest schemes. 'I work an average of twenty hours a day seven days a week as anyone living or working around me will confirm,' he asserted, randomly, in the middle of page 3. 'The secret of this is that I do not require much sleep – two hours at the most and just one if my sex life is right, which incidentally it hasn't been for some time now!' I noticed this advice popping up in letters to everyone from the Archbishop of Canterbury to his dentist.

Reading all this, I suspected Colonel B had got things backwards. Rather than thinking how much smoking and sex he needed to cure his mania, he could have wondered how best to devote his energies to something consistent with his temperament. To be sure, he might be difficult to live with, but the same can be said of many people. If he left the world with a series of new rose specimens, who could say he was a failure, any more than van Gogh was with his *Starry Night*?

22

Larry Tries to Force Georgia to Be His Accomplice

Ay, there's the rub;
For in that sleep of death what dreams may come
When we have shuffled off this mortal coil
           William Shakespeare, *Hamlet* (Act III, Scene 1)

I had a few passing thoughts about how best Dad might adapt to the world, or vice versa, but my ill-considered ideas suffered from the fact that I was focused on Larry and some thirty other people facing execution. Indeed, the best I could manage for Larry was periodic visits to try to prevent him from doing something self-destructive.

'Why don't they set me a date?' Larry complained on one visit, after a briefer discussion of the basketball season than normal. He was staring at the corner of the visiting room. The right side of his temple throbbed perceptibly.

'Your guess is as good as mine,' I said, honestly for once. 'They normally do. I guess they just haven't.'

'If you're my lawyer, you need to do what I want and get one set,' Larry said, half-heartedly. He knew I would no more get him a date than he would rat out one of his cellmates. He had written to the Attorney General – the chief prosecutor for the state of Georgia – asking how he should go about getting himself executed. He copied me in. He then sent me a copy of the AG's reply, attaching it to a one-sentence letter – 'Look what these idiots said!' It was strong language for Larry, who hardly ever called people names, unless he felt they were snitches.

He had received a form reply. The Attorney General, the

letter said, was placed in a position of conflict and could not give him legal advice. If Larry wanted to know how to get himself executed, he should consult his own lawyer. I felt sure that someone would soon wake up in the prosecutor's office.

When I next saw him, I told Larry that Judge Castellani might set a date any day now, and he affected satisfaction. I believed this to be the truth, but I was wrong. The phoney war continued. I received an official-looking letter in the mail on most days, and I thought each might bear a warrant of execution. None came.

Larry grew frustrated at the prosecution. 'Bring my trial transcripts down with you, and I will point out what they got wrong,' he wrote. 'Come on Tuesday.'

It was a breakthrough, at last, precipitated by the very people who wanted him to die. He said he would help me to prove what truly happened. I could not go on the day that he appointed, because I had to be in Mississippi through Thursday, but I sent one of our students down to reassure him that I would be there as soon as I could. She took him a copy of his entire trial record to start reviewing it with him.

I drove down to the prison on Friday, the day after I got back from Mississippi, parking in the normal place and walking past the ranks of white prison vehicles to the base of the guard tower. Today there was sunshine, and it was a guard who knew me by sight, so I did not have to shout the spelling of my name over and over before I was admitted. I felt a momentary discomfort being called in before the queue of non-legal visitors. I had nothing but a pen and a pad of paper to record Larry's thoughts. I strode along the fading squares of linoleum, mopped incessantly by a trusted prisoner, to the stairway at the end. Up the twenty steps, past the supercilious photographs of the warden and his team, to the next metal detector. It was the guard with a hunched back. She was as kindly as she felt she could get away with. She rolled the invisible ink on my left wrist and waved me onwards.

The guard in the next cubicle twisted the knob that opened the first gate, and gestured peremptorily at the ultraviolet scanner in front of him. I put my wrist under it and noticed that they had stamped 'Tuesday' on a Friday – I laughed to myself, and decided I would tell Larry I had actually come on Tuesday as he had instructed. Another twist on a knob and the second gate opened into the visitation waiting area. I knew it would be the best part of an hour, but I was happy to be seeing Larry on a positive note.

I waited. I waited. Eventually a guard came over to me. Larry refused to come out.

The guards would never tell you why. When I got back to the office, I was still wondering. Perhaps, I hoped, he had simply been taken by surprise at the visit, and had not been willing to see me without a shave and his normal soupçon of cheap cologne.

His letter arrived two days later. 'You blew your chance,' he wrote, 'when you did not come down last Tuesday. I gave you your chance. Now, nothing's going to stop me from getting this over with. Sorry! Larry.'

'Sorry!' from Larry; 'Have fun!' from Dad – the auto-sign-off to almost any letter, no matter what it said. It did not dissolve my frustration. Didn't he know I couldn't just drop all my other clients, each of them facing death? Yet salting the irritation came the guilt. It was surely my fault. I had sent him a copy of his transcript to read alone in his cell, reminding him of his honour – his commitment to dying – and allowing his demons to convince him with every page that he deserved to die. If I had been there, we could have glossed over that part; without someone to defend Larry from himself, he was doomed to self-loathing and despair.

Later he wrote to the judge. 'Dear Judge Castellani, the reason why I'm writing: I didn't want to ask you but would you please sign the "death warrant"? I'm really sorry I have to ask you 'cause I know this is going to be a struggle with you. I forgive you but when I die I hope you'll ask God to forgive you. But knowing the person you are I know you will. Thank you for your time. I'm sorry! – Larry.'

A part of me hoped that the judge would just ignore the letters, too, or lose them in his in-tray. I had other things to do at the time. I just did not need to be fighting the Attorney General, the courts and Larry all together right now. But Judge Castellani responded efficiently:

WHEREAS the jury imposed a sentence of death upon Larry Lonchar, and

WHEREAS there are no pending challenges to said sentence, or apparent impediment to it being carried out,

IT IS HEREBY ORDERED that the Warden carry out said execution at any time between noon on March 21, 1991, and noon on March 28, 1991.

DONE, this the Eighth day of March, 1991.

Robert J. Castellani, Judge

I visited Larry a couple of times. He had crossed his Rubicon, and was now quite willing to meet. He was immovable. I visited him as a friend, to keep the door open. Without his permission to file papers, our options were dramatically curtailed. And I had more profound questions. Was it the right thing to do, to stop someone from dying to escape the horrible conditions of Georgia's death row? And how far could I go to bring him back on board? The first round had been quite easy, his better nature convincing him to go forward, not wanting to waste my work.

I talked to other people to try to identify my obligation.

'Honestly, Clive, I don't know why you got yourself this Lonchar case!' said one of my colleagues in the office, exasperated. 'There are 130 people on death row in Georgia, 3,600 around the country who want your help, and you have to choose someone who doesn't!'

It was a fair point, yet somehow I felt Larry's case was my ultimate duty; he was not just hated by society, he hated himself. I was just not sure what that duty was.

It was a new feeling for me to be unsure – the privately educated tend to be instilled with an unrealistic sense of certainty. The law was no guide. I had dubbed the rule they taught in law school the 'Bad Samaritan': no citizen has a legal obligation to help someone else get out of trouble that they put themselves in, even accidentally. In the US, if you are a bystander on the banks of a river and a child falls in, you have no legal obligation to jump in to the rescue. You could be jailed for taking fifty cents from someone, but suffer no legal consequence for failing to make a minimal effort to save a life. That was obviously wrong, but I was not sure what was right. My unscientific poll of people around me suggested that most people do think about taking their own lives: studies showed that more women than men seriously contemplate it; people tend to have a preferred method in their minds – facts that surprised me. I had never pondered taking my own life for a moment.

How did my half-formed theories of euthanasia slot in? My mother had always said she did not want to be a burden. I had the sense that if she had a terminal illness where there was nothing medicine could do to alleviate the pain, and she announced that she wanted to go to Dignitas, I would get her there. Larry currently had a terminal illness – a death sentence. The long-term odds of getting him out of that predicament were good, if only he would play ball. His secondary terminal ailment was life in prison. That was trickier. The Georgia Diagnostic and Classification Center was – Larry would have insisted – in Dante's Seventh Circle of Hell, reserved for those addicted to violence. Ironically, Larry would be stuck with them: the middle ring of the same circle was peopled by those who had taken their own lives, transformed into gnarled trees with harpies gnawing at them.

Logically, the suffering of prison was curable – we just had to heed Dostoevsky and recognise that, at most, we have the right to send people to prison as a punishment, rather than to be further punished once there. Yet I was not going to be able to overhaul the Georgia prison system to suit Larry. I struggled to work out a theory that could guide me with him.

Eventually, I drew a clear line for myself the way I always had – one of the great appeals of defending people on death row for me was that the execution of my clients could never be right, no matter what they had done; it was black and white. Similarly, I decided that I had better do anything I could that was legal to stop Larry's self-destruction. The only route available was to argue that he was mentally incompetent. The law viewed the debate, again, as a question of whether his election – suicide by electric chair – was a sure-fire sign of 'mental illness', or an irrational decision by a sane mind.

We would need a 'next friend' since Larry would not sign the papers himself. This was a mechanism where someone who was mentally incompetent, or who was being coerced into an involuntary decision to die, could have another person stand in for him and bring an appeal on his behalf. It would need to be someone close to him, who was willing to swear that Larry was incapable of making his own rational decision. It would be a declaration of open war against him, and all chance of ever regaining his trust and cooperation might be forever lost. So far, while I had continually argued with him, and worked hard to get him to agree to my course of action, I had not split with him in public.

Larry would have the vast yet unimaginative power of the state on his side, as he said he wanted to die, and the state would be keen to help him have his wish. This meant we who were trying to stop him from dying might win a few skirmishes (fortunately most prosecutors are not very good at their job), but we would likely lose the war in the end. The only way for us to ultimately prevail would be to get Larry signed back onto our team.

I went in to see him, with only a few days to go before he would die. I knew I had to tell him what I was doing and why – basically because I cared about him.

'Ain't no friend of mine gonna ever say in court I need to live,' Larry said. Here, he was wrong. There were a number of willing candidates, including his mother, Elsie. I knew I could talk her into it. Although he believed he had let her down and was the cause of all her sorrows, she felt the same way about him. But the upcoming battle would be a long one, through batteries of psychiatrists, and she would not last the course. His father, Milan, would also ultimately agree to play the part, but he might be unpredictable in both his attitudes and his sobriety. That left his siblings, and any of them – Chooch, Paul or sister Chris – would agree. Whoever volunteered, or was anointed, would have to be strong enough to accept Larry's wrath. In the end we chose Chris. She had a shoulder to lean on – her husband, Terry – and she lived in Florida, which gave her the chance to retire a safer distance than the brothers, who both now lived within close visiting range of the prison.

Larry spoke almost warmly of the execution that was now only a few days away. It would be a release, he said – the only way he would ever escape the torment of prison.

Mike Mears agreed to represent Chris as 'next friend' while I tried to remain Larry's lawyer – to avoid burning the bridge to him. Mike had become a close friend since moving into my house sixteen months before when he had marriage problems, and he was still there. He came up poor, on the same street as Elvis Presley in Tupelo, before his family moved to Duck Hill, Mississippi. I visited his parents there, with the Confederate battle flag in the living room and guns littered through the house. There was a lump in the mattress in the spare bedroom – an Uzi, it transpired. Mike's father gleefully demonstrated its potential for protecting Middle Mississippi from the communist threat, raking various washing machines and dishwashers piled up in the backyard.

Mike had made it to the American Dream. He escaped Mississippi via the military, and then moved to teaching school in Georgia. A law degree later, he became a partner in the very proper firm of McCurdy & Candler, before being elected mayor of Decatur for ten years. Mayor Mears had hit a midlife crisis when he had first been roped into a capital case at the firm. He found that the law had a purpose. After his third capital case made the local newspaper, his white-collar partners asked him whether he would allow them to buy him out of the business. He was now short on cash, but happy persecuting prosecutors. He was the ideal person to represent Chris. The long-term prospects of her cause seemed hopeless, but Mike was happier tilting at windmills than was Don Quixote.

With three days left before he was due to die, the prison saw an opportunity to make it far more difficult to talk Larry round: they said he did not want a lawyer, so I could not visit him. His depression, they realised, gave them another strategic advantage: they refused him medication. It would be easier to usher him into the chair if he remained utterly miserable.

In years gone by, stopping a 'date' in Georgia had been easier. The execution was set for a specific time and day, and if you were sufficiently verbose in the legal pleadings, and waited to file papers until the eleventh hour, a stay might be forthcoming simply because the judges did not have time to read everything. They had long since got wise to this: the executioner was allowed a week in which to kill the prisoner – the 'Execution Window'.

The warden would set the execution for 7 p.m. on the first

day, and the defence might get a brief stay, but even if the execution was delayed a day or two it could still be carried out before the seventh moon rose.

Larry's dance with death began on the afternoon of Thursday 21 March.

Mike filed Chris's 'next friend' petition alleging Larry's inability to make a rational decision, and a hearing was immediately set before a state judge, Hal Craig. Craig had heard many capital appeals and denied virtually every one, though I found it difficult to dislike him. Some of his colleagues were just plain mean. Not Craig. He was clean-cut and short, an abbreviated version of an all-American, generally pleasant and polite with the occasional temper tantrum that seemed to stem from the frustration of not knowing what he was doing. This was a positive quality. The worst elected judges are smart and mean: they are motivated to kill the client, and they know how to do it. In contrast, at the end of every hearing, Craig would retire to chambers to deliberate with himself. Goodness knows what he did back there – his office was rather sparse, and there was not even a dartboard. He would then emerge with the same answer: *Denied*. He composed his own opinions, and the incomprehensible quality of his prose made an appeal far more fruitful since he made so many mistakes.

It was already Thursday morning when we filed, and Judge Craig would likely have denied our application on that same day but for the state's request for time to respond – the next of many moves in the macabre game where the state helped us to keep Larry alive. In the end, he rescheduled a hearing for the following Tuesday, the 26th, when the parties were meant to bring in their evidence. This was a victory from our perspective, since this whittled away most of the allotted week before we had a chance to lose the first round of appeals. Yet there was a problem – the perennial problem – for the defence: how could we present any kind of case when we had no money? While the state could hire any available expert, the defence was not even allowed the pittance required to issue subpoenas so that witnesses would attend the hearing. The state had various experts evaluate Larry – a psychiatrist, and more than one psychologist. They had the prison take Larry to their hospital facilities to conduct neurological tests. For much of this time I did not even know where he was.

When I saw him just before the hearing began, Larry told me how he had tired of the state's experts. He talked about it matter-of-factly, but I was encouraged – if he really wanted to die, he would have cooperated with them. He had wanted to see the play-offs of the NCAA college basketball season, so he'd refused to take any more tests and demanded to be taken back to his cell on death row to watch what was scheduled to be his last basketball game. It was still only the quarter-final round of the tournament.

We started the hearing at nine that Tuesday morning. At the outset, Warden Walter Zant announced that he planned to execute Larry early the next morning, so our frantic filibuster began. We did not have an expert to call to testify, but on the optimistic promise that we would eventually be able to come up with some funds, we had been able to get an affidavit from a well–respected psychiatrist from Yale University, who had seen Larry and diagnosed him as bipolar, manic-depressive – more often down than up, and desperate to die in the depths of his frequent and enduring depressions. Meanwhile, Mike was the master of taking a one-hour hearing and making it last all day. I still have no idea where he came up with all the things to ask, making everything seem fresh and somehow relevant. There was no stopping him – wind him up, push him towards the courtroom, and Mike was the Energizer Bunny in the battery adverts: he would keep going, and going, and going.

The prosecution began to call their perennial parade of experts culled from the state hospitals. Everyone agreed that Larry was depressed, but the doctors tried to play it down as situational – of course he was, he was on death row. They insisted on this at great length, in varying degrees, as Mike took them through what little they knew for hours on end. By lunchtime, Mike looked like he could keep them at it for the rest of the week. Five hours later, we came to the end of the working day. Judge Craig said he would continue all night if need be. Eight o'clock came and went, and Mike was still going. The hands moved towards nine o'clock, and even Mike was running out of ideas. The prosecution had finally figured him out, and chose not to call anyone else for him to torment. We had to come up with something ourselves. Mike extracted a five-minute break out of the judge. We huddled over what to do.

Perhaps we could have one witness – me. Who knew more about Larry's oscillations? We would pose the kind of dilemma that the judge would hate: anything I said would fall under the attorney–client privilege, and could not be disclosed without Larry's consent. So I took the stand and I invoked Larry's rights for him. Judge Craig was perplexed. He turned to Larry and asked him if he would waive his privilege. Larry never wanted to offend anyone, and immediately said yes. The judge was happy, but we had considered that possibility: I said that since, in my opinion, he was not competent to decide to die, I could not accept that he was capable of waiving his legal rights. Judge Craig was confused again. Finally, after much debate, he refused to allow me to testify. Until he decided that Larry was competent, he could not hear my evidence that Larry was not competent: Yossarian would have been proud of the catch-22. Larry whispered appreciatively to me when I got off the stand. He had enjoyed the show. He always did enjoy a good gambit.

We could divine no other way to keep the brakes on the steam train. Judge Craig retired to 'deliberate' with himself for what he deemed an acceptable time and then ruled against us on grounds that Larry's decision to die was totally rational. The execution could proceed the next morning, less than twelve hours away from us now. Larry walked with that stiff back of his out of the courtroom, a guard on either side, his wrists shackled in front of him, his leg irons rattling along the wooden floor.

'. . . Later, Clive,' he said as he went by.

The next movement of the dance was on. We had to get to the Georgia Supreme Court before morning. Rushing back to the office, Mike and I stayed up most of the night together assembling a stay petition. We delivered it to the court early. There was no way they could really read it all before the execution deadline, but I was confident they would refuse to hear it, and pass the buck to the federal courts. We started to ready the papers for the next appeal.

Larry would now be almost ready for execution – they would soon be shaving his head, for better contact with the sponge that connected the electrode on the helmet to his brain. They would also shave his shin to have a clean point of contact for the other electrode, so that the 2,000 volts could run unimpeded between his leg and his skull. Every now and then, as I typed his petition, wild thoughts would intrude. I remembered my physics A level – voltage is equal to the current times the resistance. Someone once worked out that a human body, with one electrode on the head and one on the ankle, creates roughly 2,000 ohms in resistance, so 2,000 volts would produce a current of just one amp, but surprisingly that would be enough to kill a person. Albeit as the body is cooked . . .

Then the impending deadline would drag my mind back. I typed frantically, moving paragraphs from this document to that.

Miraculously, the Georgia Supreme Court issued a stay. They would need several weeks to study the case, they said. So we had avoided this date with the executioner – although the state tried vainly to persuade the court to change its mind and allow the killing to go ahead.

I went to see Larry as soon as I was permitted. Now there was no execution date, the prison let me in even though from their perspective Larry still did not want a lawyer.

He was overtly manic. He was angry. I had expected that. Astoundingly, his ire was not directed at me.

'Did you see that? M---a---n!' he said loudly. He put several syllables of frustration in the word – a crescendo, then a trailing off. I had never seen Larry this agitated. The guard beyond the yellow metal gate looked up at us. I nodded at him over Larry's shoulder, to head off any intervention.

'Did you see that?' he repeated. 'That woman . . . that woman, a sister or something.' He was having difficulty completing a sentence. Slowly, he explained what had happened on Wednesday, when his execution had been stayed. He had been a spectator watching his own funeral. Several of the victims' family members had gone on television that day saying how much they wanted to see him die, and how furious they were that they had been denied their pleasure. Larry had been flagellated by his own conscience. He had kept on watching. Then one of them said how she had spent so much money on a new dress, because she knew she would be on camera as they came out from the execution. It was unfair, she was saying, that she had been put to that expense, only to be denied her moment on the retribution catwalk. Larry's penitence gave way to anger: to have his death treated as a pretext for a shopping expedition! For a moment he wanted to live, if only to prevent the degradation of this kind of death.

Larry talked about re-joining his own team. Yet the change was only transient, and he soon slipped back into depression. He needed more than a momentary catharsis; he needed the promise of a lifetime of hope.

23

The Justin Shaffer Case

Support Mrs Thatcher! Royalists demand return of the rope!
                                                    Henry Root

David Utter and I had worked together in Atlanta, spending
many evenings in the local pub. We thought we could do more
of the same in New Orleans, the best city to live in if one was
consigned to the Death Belt, which was where we had to be.
Repairing most evenings to the Acme Oyster House on Iber-
ville Street in the French Quarter, we planned to change the
emphasis of our work – it was time to stop the death row dam
from filling up, rather than merely using our thumbs to prevent
it from bursting. We would focus almost entirely on trials rather
than appeals. We concocted a sibilant abbreviation – the
LCAC – for a stupid name, designed to disguise what we did
and avoid some of the bomb threats: the Louisiana Crisis Assistance Center.

   One of the first cases we had was to defend Carl Hall in
Orleans Parish. Carl and Cathy Hall had two kids who he
insisted should be called Carl Jr and Carlita. Carl was self-
obsessed. He and Cathy had separated but their relationship
continued in turbulence. Carl saw her in a white, two-door
Oldsmobile Cutlass Supreme with a man called Hubert Steib.
His rival's car was an important status symbol, as significant to
Carl's loss of control as seeing his wife with another man. He
pulled alongside Steib's vehicle and began firing through the
open windows. Steib valiantly attempted to push Cathy down,
and was himself shot in the arm. Carl ran out of bullets. Steib

crawled out of the car, telling Cathy to run for it. He dashed for an alley where, turning back, he realised that Carl had no interest in him.

Cathy managed to slide out, but the car started rolling and ran over her leg, breaking it. Carl ran around and beat her with the empty pistol, then pulled a knife.

'Please, Carl!' Cathy begged. 'Don't kill me.'

'Bitch!' Carl shouted. 'I told you not to play with me like this! . . . I told you not to mess with me like this!'

Carl stabbed her and then jumped back into his car and drove off. Sadly, she was dead before she made it to the hospital. The police swiftly issued a warrant for Carl's arrest, and he turned himself in. At the first trial, he received the standard, derisory defence from a drunken lawyer, and was sentenced to death. The Supreme Court of Louisiana reversed his case for a new trial because of errors in jury selection, and David and I agreed to do it. I felt relatively sure we would get him convicted of the lesser offence of manslaughter – he could still get a hefty term, up to forty years, but it would not be death. Indeed, it was the first heat-of-passion case I'd had since I had got furious and lost control of myself with Cristiana in Atlanta. I hated to think that I should view that incident in any kind of positive light, but at least I had a better idea of what was – or was not – going through Carl's mind at the time, which made me better able to present the truth to the jury.

The case was to be tried in Division I of the Mussolini Mausoleum – Orleans Parish Criminal District Court – the massive 1930s building on the corner of Tulane and Broad avenues, a venue of much injustice. The state had called in a 'Sanity Commission' to assess Carl for any mental health defence. This was a fly-by farce. A 'forensic psychiatrist' – a grizzled white man who spent more of his day leaning on the bar at Lafitte's Blacksmith – came into the courtroom and sat in the jury box with the defendant. There, he conducted his 'evaluation', whereupon he issued a report, which was all of two or three sentences.

The doctor was being paid by the state, and so his report inevitably opined that Carl was totally sane, wholly responsible for his actions, a sociopath who had no conscience. The doctor had spent too much time behind a glass of bourbon to read the diagnostic manual, or he would have used the modern label, ASPD. I had to prepare for this man to take the stand and relay his professional conclusions to a jury. At the LCAC, we made up for a lack of resources with some brilliant young volunteers who would do the large part of the work for which I got the credit. I set one of them to researching every instance where this charlatan had ever testified.

She went down to the Supreme Court on Loyola Avenue, and assembled a stack of thirty or forty homicide transcripts where he had taken the stand. There was a stark pattern. When he was hired by the prosecution, the defendant was invariably a young African American man who he maintained was a sociopath who knew right from wrong, and should be duly punished. When he was hired by the other side, the defendant had to have money, which was generally the prerogative of a middle-class white male who, he decided, was suffering from manic depression. Each time, in his view, this meant that his well-heeled white client met the 1843 M'Naghten Rule, still in operation in Louisiana: the accused did not understand the difference between right and wrong, or did not understand that what he was doing was wrong.

I pondered whether to label him a quack. I settled on 'mountebank'. I liked the Italian derivation, from *monta in banco*, describing the way that a salesman used to get up on a bench to address his potential customers. I knew we would have a sympathetic jury in Orleans Parish, and that our survey of this man and his ridiculous racism would not go down well with them. I anticipated slapping down each transcript on the dark oak of the witness stand, systematically checking off each race-driven diagnosis on the blackboard. This alone would, I knew, save Carl from any death sentence.

A capital trial is the greatest laxative known to humanity. The moment I approached one without being nervous, I would know I was in the wrong business. Preparing for Carl's case, I took long walks along the quiet Mississippi River in the early morning, thinking of the best approach. One morning I had a sudden revelation: the shrink was a fraud, to be sure, but in one respect he was right. When my father was manic, he simply didn't know right from wrong. Had he been prosecuted for child abuse when he gave me £200 and told me it was time for me to make it on my own at the age of seven, Dad should have been found 'insane' even under the archaic definition of insanity in M'Naghten.

Carl was acquitted of capital murder, and convicted, as I had hoped, of the lesser offence of manslaughter. Yet for me, personally, this was a seminal moment. I had an insight into my father that had eluded me for many years, such that my life now made sense. Dad was truly not Bad – he might be a brilliant Cambridge graduate, but he was so out of touch with reality that he was not guilty, by reason of insanity.

If a mountebank psychiatrist could get that much right, then surely we could muddle our way towards a sensible way to approach 'responsibility'. I would no longer blame Dad for the decisions he made. I would have to look solely at how I could help make his life better.

Justin Shaffer's trial was a difficult experience.

Thursday, 14 March 1991 was the day Justin was alleged to have killed Rachel Marshall. We were forced to trial just eleven months later, on 3 February 1992. I had already tried one capital case in January – Otis Grimsley in Alabama. The trial had ended the week before – in a hung jury, with seven black jurors for acquittal on all charges, five whites for conviction for capital murder. From its headquarters in Chicago, the American Bar Association had issued an edict that the maximum number of capital cases any lawyer should have at any time was two, a luxury we could not afford in the Deep South: I had thirty now, and at least five would go to trial in the first eight months. It was the year when I spent 270 days in court in six different states from Louisiana to Florida and up to Virginia, and it just about did for me, Justin Shaffer's case more than most.

Justin's judge was perfectly amicable in a prosecutorial sort of way, and she called the medics when I started having heart problems towards the closing argument at the culpability phase. They brought a portable electrocardiogram into the courtroom and tested me while I lay down on one of the audience pews. The case had been high on pressure, short on time and resources.

By far the greatest stressor had been Dad.

It was all my fault. I had an ill-thought-out theory about Dad, ultimately a solipsism: I thought he might find satisfaction in my world. His primary problem, so went my theory, was that he was always trying to make enormous sums of money. He would have an idea, he would charge forward, but nothing would translate into reality, the ideas left strewn in his wake – along with the battered people who had been caught up, momentarily, in his enthusiasm. Dad could never hope to meet his own expectations, let alone those of others.

Meanwhile, I had muddled my way into a life I loved, and I thought it might suit Dad, since I shared much of his temperament. I had been propelled by the nonconformist zeal I had inherited from him, and also by the fear that I would end up in the same vortex of capitalism that left the stud and every SAPPSA project in shambles. I was finally clear on why I represented people on death row: I looked around the world for the most hated people I could find, and got between them and the ones doing the hating. This made everything simple, black and white.

I faced calamity daily; I made mistakes daily. However, unless I did the initial trial, I could blame my disasters on a number of external causes (at least on a psychological level). While I was astounded that a justice system could allow someone as callow as me to hold life and death in the balance, the truth was that someone in Larry's position had no alternative. The US Supreme Court had held – in 1989, in *Murray* v. *Giarratano* – that a prisoner on death row had no right to counsel funded by the state, which meant that everyone was dependent upon a do-gooder zealot like me who would take the case on without being paid.

All this worked for me. I realised that it was a self-protective mechanism that I was using to stave off the possibility of being a 'failure', but it seemed like a good one, since it simultaneously fulfilled my mother's first directive: life is all about helping people who are worse off than we are. As she used to say, if everyone did that, we would all be better off.

So I set about solving Dad's world for him, with much the same blindness that he would have shown. It might have worked out if I had been his careers adviser in 1942, but there was no real chance that he was going to enter a profession where his son had already staked out some territory. But I never thought about that. Instead, I invited him over to see how my life worked, thinking that perhaps he would get into something similar, that would allow him to devote his immense energy to people who needed it (rather than to SAPPSA). I was merely doing what I always did so well with Dad – failing to think it through, and therefore setting up the next disaster.

Dad showed up in Biloxi in January 1992, a month before Justin Shaffer's trial. Justin's father, Colonel Paul Shaffer, a US military pathologist, had kindly offered him a place to stay. Paul was a gaunt and sombre man, much more middle-class than most of my clients' parents, and his profession gave him a good understanding of some of the issues in the case. We had to deal with a particularly notorious forensic pathologist from the Gulf Coast, and Paul's insights were helpful. Understandably, though, he was all emotion when it came to his son.

I did not have much time to prepare, and I belatedly worked out that my brilliant idea that my field of endeavour might appeal to Dad was going to prove a serious distraction, just when I did not need it. Rather, I hoped that perhaps Paul and Dad would keep each other occupied, and let me get on with the job. We had dinner at Paul's house one evening, the bright orange Thousand Island salad dressing clashing with the red-checked tablecloth.

'My immediate thinking, you see,' Dad remarked airily, to both of us, 'based on what you are already doing, is to set up a whole series of parallel structures like your public defence service . . . except that they would be self-activating and entirely self-motivating . . . I mean, designed to do things which the present system is patently failing to do.'

I interjected that, while nobody could disagree with him, our immediate problem was to try to extricate Justin from his current predicament.

Dad's sojourn in Mississippi set him on a rapid rise again. He went home briefly, filling Mum in on what a disaster I was. 'My sister Jean and Clive are so alike that I find it almost uncanny dealing with them!' he said. 'I mean, they are both what we in the trade call well-meaning do-gooders . . . the type of person who causes far more trouble in the world than an outright rogue!' He assured her that he would make sure I did my job properly.

Before he came back to Mississippi, there was more excitement. He learned that he might have a claim to be lord of the manor in Cheveley, the pointless title that his father had bought for £10 back in the 1940s to go with the stud. Somehow, in the bankruptcy, nobody had thought to foreclose on that.

'I am excited by the lordship of the manor!' he told Mum. 'I mean, as you know, I have always seen myself as a Knight of the Round Table with a touch of the Don Quixote, so I can see a number of ways in which the lordship could be useful.'

Alongside the authority to dictate to the locals where they might plant trees on the village green, the second risible power bestowed upon the lordship was the right to raise a private army from the serfs of Cheveley.

'I might raise a force,' Dad continued. He immediately sat down to write to Ralph Howell MP, a right-wing Tory in Norfolk, whose main parliamentary proposals included compulsory national service, the reintroduction of the death penalty, and stronger controls on immigration. Dad proposed that he should raise a peacekeeping brigade for the UN from the village. I think a brigade generally comprises some 2,000 soldiers. The village population was then 1,900, a number of whom were pensioners, residents of the Cheveley Evergreen Club where Mum was a trustee. Not many people would be left behind to prune the trees Dad might allow to be planted.

Dad then returned to Mississippi. He again stayed with Colonel Shaffer; I stayed in a motel along the railroad tracks, with deafening whistles all through the night. After a week-long trial, with me almost in hospital, fortunately Justin was found not guilty of capital murder, but he was convicted of simple murder. Dad was in the courtroom for the first couple of days, but was aghast at both the legal process and the glaring ineptitude of his son. He stormed out and took a bus up to Jackson, the capital. Eloquent and persuasive as ever, he talked his way into the governor's mansion, and sat down for a glass of iced tea with the person in charge of the state.

From then on, I have only his report of the conversation.

'I have a difficult time believing, Governor, what is going on in your state, down there in Biloxi,' he began. 'I mean, first, you have to see the way the system is operating, or not operating.'

I imagined the governor nodding, non-committal.

'But the real problem,' he continued, 'is the death penalty. Not your use of it – of course you have the right to use it . . .'

Now I thought the governor probably raised an eyebrow in surprise at this European, who would normally be expected to deliver a lecture on the barbarism of capital punishment.

'Of course you should . . . of course you should. But you see, you should do it now. Justin Shaffer . . . he could start again. Reincarnation . . . I mean, I'm sure you understand . . . it's a scientific fact, it's the way he will have another chance, and not mess up with drugs, like he did this time.'

I was not sure what the governor thought at this point.

'And while you're about it, that son of mine,' Dad reported saying, in total seriousness, 'I mean, you might just execute him as well, and give him another chance.'

I had recently read *The Henry Root Letters*, William Donaldson's publication of spoofs sent to people who take themselves too seriously. The fictional Henry Root would write a missive that was outrageous for its chauvinism or its UKIP-esque racism, congratulating a public figure who somehow exemplified a 'Make Britain Great Again' spirit. He would often include money to support the person's good works – 'Here's a pound!' – with the same enthusiasm as Dad signed off with 'Have fun!' The inclusion of a pound note was a cunning ruse as it made people write back, either to thank him for what was perceived to be a political donation or to return the money. A small minority chided him for his prejudice; fewer still guessed it was a joke and replied in kind; the majority wrote a pompous letter that did its author no favours.

One of my favourites was addressed to Her Majesty the Queen (and her husband, the 'Duke of Normandy'): 'I surmise that as a mother you will be no less concerned than Mrs Root is about this once great nation's collapse in terms of moral leadership.' He went on to suggest that in addition to all the openings Her Majesty was obliged to carry out, she might consider closing a few things – like the National Liberal Club,

BBC2 and subversive publications like the *New Statesman*. He signed off heartily: 'Support Mrs Thatcher! Royalists demand return of the rope!'

I hated listening to Dad telling me the story of his travels. I imagined everyone laughing at him. The governor of Mississippi had probably been wondering whether Henry Root had come for a glass of iced tea. My plan to introduce Dad to capital defence work had not gone as I had hoped. I would have to think of something better.

As was generally the case, we parted on good terms when I saw Dad off at the airport. He left me his assessment:

> The plane takes off as I depart
> And leave behind two weeks of joy!
> His dreams fulfilled – in mind and heart –
> The grown-up version of the boy!

As ever, I was not sure what to make of the note. As ever, I was busy, so I pushed my failure to convert Dad to the background and got on with life.

My year continued: I had to try Otis Grimsley's case a second time – he was acquitted of capital murder but convicted of robbery. One of the African American jurors apologised for the conviction afterwards, saying that his fellow jurors had compromised with the white members of the panel, as nobody wanted Otis sent back to Henry County where they thought he might be lynched. Then came Joe Beauville: we had got his death sentence reversed and he was convicted at retrial of simple murder. The district attorney got so angry at the judge, who made one ruling against him, that he went into the judge's chambers and pissed on his carpet. Nothing came of it; I wondered what would happen to me if I did that. The fifth capital trial of my year was Sam Johnson's in Vicksburg: I called Sheriff

Lloyd 'Goon' Jones as a witness on a motion to dismiss the charges because of the general aura of racism in the case against Sam. Jones admitted that he no longer called black men 'niggers'; now he called them 'coloured boys'. The four black jurors voted for life, and that was enough to avoid death.

24

Larry's Rational Suicide

When Irrational is deemed to be Rational in the name of
Power, Madness reigns Supreme.

The issue before Federal District Judge Jack Camp was whether
Larry Lonchar was competent to decide that he wanted to die.
I had hope. Camp struck me as a reasonable person, and unlike
many judges he had some real-world experience: he had been
brought up on a farm in Coweta County and been drafted into
Vietnam right after the Tet Offensive. He later became a lawyer, inspired by *To Kill a Mockingbird*, and had defended criminal
cases: when he won one murder trial on a self-defence theory,
he ended up between his client and the victim's widow as she
came down the aisle of the courtroom, angrily brandishing a
butcher's knife.

He was unvaryingly polite in the Southern style. He sat high
up on his federal bench, with his shock of white hair. He had
found the state court hearing inadequate, partly due to the testimony back then of Dr Robert Storms. Storms was a
psychologist who had achieved local notoriety when he diagnosed a dog. According the official letter he sent to the
municipal judge on that case, the animal met the M'Naghten
criteria under Georgia law when he ran out and bit the postman, because he did not know right from wrong. Every dog is
normally allowed one bite, yet animals evaluated by Storms
would be allowed to chew on postmen ad infinitum, always
found not guilty by reason of canine insanity. Storms had

deemed Larry, on the other hand, fit to be executed, and he had testified to this in the state court proceedings.

Unknown to Mike Mears and me at the time, Dr Storms was not actually the psychologist who had evaluated Larry. That task had gone to Dr David Pritchard – but Larry, with his eternal ambivalence, had elected to watch a college basketball game that afternoon on television rather than cooperate. When Dr Pritchard had appeared at the courthouse and told the prosecutors that ethically he could say nothing about Larry's mental state, he had been sent away to prevent Mike and me from running into him and perhaps calling him as our own witness. Later, when he read about the case in the newspaper, he learned that Dr Storms had testified. He was incensed, and called me to say that he had made a complaint with the state psychological commission. Dr Storms had not, he said, conducted any meaningful evaluation of Larry, and it was unethical for him to pretend that he had.

A fresh hearing had to be held, at which three doctors were to give evidence. This time it would be in the ugly modern federal building, up on the twenty-first floor in a large room without windows. Behind the judge's throne was the flag of the United States with an eagle rising like a phoenix from the wall, inscribed 'In God We Trust'. Judge Camp listened patiently to a number of experts testifying about Larry. Once more, Mike Mears had the job of keeping the witnesses going for three days.

The first was Dr Everett Kuglar. I had known him across several cases, and I had seen him speak to juries; he treated us all like cherished grandchildren. He was the director of the state psychiatric hospital and was prepared to go the extra mile when he felt that the prosecution was acting on the basis of politics rather than good sense. Even though he was on the other side today, I liked the man.

Larry and I sat together admiring Mike's technique. It was a bizarre setting. Larry supposedly wanted to die, but he was beside me, whispering disparaging remarks about the prosecutors as Mike and I battled his wishes. It was as if it lent his fragile sense of ego a little validation, though not enough to make him want to live on. Mike swept his grey hair back, pulled his trousers up – a habit he had, girding himself for combat – and started pressing Dr Kuglar on cross-examination. The doctor agreed that Larry suffered from a 'mental illness', and was severely depressed. He had a personality disorder that contributed to his sense of worthlessness. 'The hallmark of this individual's personality construct is such that he will frequently make decisions that are not in his best interest,' Kuglar opined. 'He does this in a way which would essentially be characterised as self–defeating.'

The prison was still refusing Larry any therapy or medication for his illness. Mike and I had a theory, laboriously woven through the hearing: in denying Larry medication, the prison was actively the accomplice to his suicide. It has long been the law in most states, including Georgia, that to aid someone who wishes to take his own life is a criminal offence. There was a precedent where a prisoner was waiting to be hanged; a cellmate by the name of Bowen encouraged his condemned friend to kill himself before the state could get him. For cheating the government out of its just deserts, Bowen became eligible for the death penalty himself.

If Warden Zant helped Larry to commit suicide by denying medication, he should be locked up in his own prison. It was unlikely that the argument would succeed, but Zant shifted with some discomfort when we first made it. According to my own mental health manual, Zant's psychological diagnosis was 'Napoleonic asshole', and anything that made him unhappy went in the win column; Larry concurred.

Even as we were debating Larry's case in court, the nation

was being held in thrall by the tales of Dr Jack Kevorkian, who had advertised across the country his specialised assistance in euthanasia. Dr Kevorkian was viewed by some as a macabre messenger of death, by some as a hero, and by others as a media whore. The Georgia legislature had responded by strengthening the law banning helping a suicide. 'We wanted to take a stand, here and now, before Dr Kevorkian came to Georgia,' Representative Ron Crews, a Republican from Gwinnett County, had announced recently in the local paper.

There was no doubt that Larry's untreated 'mental illness' was contributing to his decision, Dr Kuglar conceded. His depression was eminently treatable. Lithium had been on the market for fifty years, and that might be reasonably effective, or there were better modern drugs. Dr Kuglar testified that Larry's treatment was medically mandated. No ethical physician would deprive a suicidal man of his medicine.

'Larry's ambivalence is rather prominent,' each of the experts agreed. 'This is someone who wants to die but doesn't want to die.' All agreed that Larry was crying out for help.

'Then there was a question about suicide,' testified Dr Davis, the second expert for the state. Dave Davis was a suave witness with a reputation for being friendly to whoever was paying his bills. With a little prompting from Mike, he was behaving himself well today. 'My question to him,' he continued, 'was did he think that by waiving his appeal rights that there was . . . that this was a kind of suicide, and Larry explained to me that, in a way, it was.'

'Would you agree,' asked Mike, reading the dilemma from a psychiatric textbook, 'that "suicide is a preventable cause of death because almost all suicide victims suffer from a treatable psychiatric disorder, and the great majority of them communicate their self–destructive intentions to those around them, including their physicians"?'

Dr Davis agreed.

'Would you also agree that "all those involved in community services must be taught about the causes, diagnosis, and treatments, about the groups at risk for suicide and how to assess and manage the person who is suicidal"?'

Dr Davis agreed again. He could not deny that Hippocrates insisted that anyone who was suicidal, and who was not otherwise terminally ill, must be treated rather than encouraged in their self-destruction.

'Dr Davis, is Larry today terminally ill?' asked Mike, several hours into his cross-examination filibuster. Judge Camp was a patient man.

'No,' he replied.

'Is the mental disorder for which you have diagnosed Larry treatable?'

'Potentially,' he confessed. Larry was potentially treatable – that was, if the state would agree to treat him; without this treatment, Larry was terminally ill and the cause of death would be electrocution. 'He is forcing the criminal justice system to become an accomplice in his own destruction, I guess that's obvious.'

'If an individual expressed a present intent to commit suicide or to self–destruct, would you have a professional responsibility to take action to prevent their self–harm?'

'Yes,' Dr Davis eventually conceded. This was really the crux of this case: if everyone agreed that Larry should be treated, why in the name of heaven was he not being given treatment? If I were to smuggle the necessary medicine into the prison, or even a different drug so Larry could voluntarily and painlessly pass out of this life, I would be arrested and locked up alongside him. The only person with the power over Larry's treatment was Warden Zant.

Now it was Dr Robert Phillips's turn to talk. He had given us the original affidavit in the state proceedings, but since we were now in federal court, we had been allowed funds for our own expert. A very well-spoken, rotund black man with unparalleled qualifications, Dr Phillips once joked that a case we had worked on together had put one of his kids through college. Nobody in our charity saw the humour, given the percentage of our annual budget we had been forced to spend. His fee was $250 for every hour out of his office, precisely fifty times my hourly wage at the time. When your client's life is at stake, it is difficult to decide when an hourly fee is too much for a valuable witness. He could be worth it – he was capable of putting everything in the best light.

'Someone walks into the emergency room at Yale New Haven Hospital and says, "I'm entertaining the notion of killing myself."' Dr Phillips posed the hypothetical, being sure to underline that he was at the premier medical school in the US. 'If it is someone who is truly clinically depressed and is at high risk for committing that act, I would probably involuntarily admit that person to the hospital in order to make a more careful determination and, if the conditions warranted, I would either voluntarily or involuntarily medicate the individual with antidepressants with the hope that the commitment to suicide would dissipate.'

Dr Kuglar and Dr Davis waffled for a while, but came down on diagnoses of depression and a personality disorder. Dr Phillips was the only one to find Larry to be bipolar. To the extent that the label was significant, Dr Phillips was clearly right: I had seen the cycles myself for several years now. The distinction, in the odd world of psychiatry, was between a psychotic illness and what some experts view as just the person's 'character', and it played into the next question: was Larry's choice 'rational' and competent? Dr Phillips said no; the others said it was.

In the end, I testified – either for Larry, or against him, it was not quite clear. I was half worried to look at him as I repeated some of the things he had told me over the months before and even during the hearing. Every few minutes, Larry had leaned over to tell me how he disagreed with the state experts' testimony, suggesting ways that we could better cross-examine them. He defied logic, helping us when we were trying to stop him from reaching the goal that he supposedly craved.

When I left the stand, Larry thanked me. He was glad I had spoken on his behalf.

Finally, silence awaited Judge Camp's decision. He was not a liberal man, but unlike many of his colleagues he was working hard to be a decent one. Camp pondered aloud the bizarre quality of the past three days. He turned to the man whose life was in the balance. 'Mr Lonchar, you have been here during the entire proceedings. And I know at times this has been uncomfortable for you, seeing your competency debated by several experts and talking about things that are personal and private in nature.'

The judge wanted to know what it was that was driving Larry to his death.

'What bothers you, Mr Lonchar?'

'I'm alive,' Larry replied in a monotone. 'That's what bothers me.'

'Well, let me ask you this: what is the effect upon you personally of the execution of your sentence?' Judge Camp was focused on one of the legal issues – what we refer to as 'competency to be executed': whether Larry understood what would happen to him when he died. It is a peculiar enquiry; Larry would, supposedly, be rational if he expressed the view that it would just be the end of him, ashes to ashes. Equally, he would be deemed competent if he suddenly converted to Christianity and said he would go to heaven, sitting at the right hand of God Himself. Yet if he were my dad, and insisted on the scientific certainty that he would come right back round after reincarnation, Judge Camp might be inclined to commit him to the state hospital. I sat with my head in my hands, wondering who in the courtroom was 'mad'.

Larry was not going to be drawn in. 'I'm not really going to go into that. What difference does it really make?'

'I want to make sure you understand, since your competence has been questioned here by experts, that the effect of execution is a final and irremediable effect, and that is that you are dead. Do you have a full understanding of that?'

'Yes, sir,' Larry said dully.

Judge Camp mentioned that the method of execution was the electric chair – with 2,000 volts passed through his brain. Larry paled, but refused to comment. I had looked into his eyes when we had discussed the chair. I knew the poor man was very afraid.

'Mr Lonchar, I would like you to tell me in your own words why you have reached the decision that you would like to waive any further appeals and accept the execution of your sentence.'

'Your Honour, there are many reasons, you know. I just . . .' I watched him, half excited that he might finally put it into words, half dreading that a well-reasoned reply would be his death warrant. Larry trailed off, almost whining. 'You know, I just feel . . . Why do I have to justify this?'

'Well . . .' The judge was not satisfied. Like Judge Castellani and the jurors before him, Judge Camp had been given great power, and he was not thrilled that he had to exercise it. He, too, might become an accomplice in Larry's self-destruction.

'This is my life!' Larry started up again, his voice rising now in sad desperation. Judge Camp had driven up from his farm that morning, and had set the hearing for a time convenient to his calendar. There was little chance he could truly comprehend Larry's life. During the hearing, Larry could not go to the toilet without the judge's permission. 'I have made this decision. Why are we even here? I don't understand this. There are many reasons, you know. One doctor testified that it is because I don't want to spend the rest of my life in prison. You know, that is his version. That's not true. I'm institutionalised. I have been incarcerated the last twenty-five years. Doing time doesn't bother me.'

If facing life in prison was not the real reason, Larry would still not give another. 'I don't feel I owe anyone all of my reasons. I know why I want to die,' he said. I wondered whether this was true. 'Nothing personal against the court or anything, there are many reasons.'

'Well, I respect your feelings in that regard, Mr Lonchar,' the judge replied. 'But I think it's a fair question—'

'Yes,' Larry interjected. Larry hated to disagree with anyone if he thought he might give offence. It was ever more surreal, a long and extremely public discussion with someone who was trying to die by suicide. The court reporter was taking down his words. The journalists were scribbling in the audience.

'You ask me why I would ask you to justify that, and I will try to tell you,' the judge continued, rubbing his chin with his hand. 'I'm going to have to make a decision here and, quite frankly, having you tell me what you considered and why you made that decision I think is a relevant enquiry to assist me in making the decision I must make.'

'If you would like to go in your chambers and off the public record,' Larry said, 'I will tell you, because there are many personal reasons, you know. But it has been embarrassing enough that all these things have been said about my family and everything.'

For a moment I wondered whether the judge would call Larry's bluff. Judge Camp was an avuncular personality, and perhaps Larry was prepared to open up to him. Yet the judge had an impossible human task, and the law did not allow him to be human. Larry's privacy ranked low in importance, and the judge was forced to say that he could not hear anything from Larry that was not on the public record.

'From the beginning, you know, I gave up,' Larry eventually mumbled on. 'You can say years ago . . . from the beginning. Even at my trial, if I would have cooperated with my defence lawyer, I'm sure I wouldn't be here . . . But I have my reasons.'

Judge Camp obviously did not want to have to make the

decision at all. He left the bench, saying he would rule as soon as he could.

Weeks later, when he gave his opinion, it was apparent that Judge Camp had been struggling. He agreed with all three doctors that Larry was ill, though he was not willing to go along with Dr Phillips's opinion that Larry should be considered bipolar.

'Mr Lonchar suffers from a mental disorder,' the judge said. 'He has suffered chronic depression for a number of years which has been correctly diagnosed as dysthymia. He also suffers from a personality disorder, which includes antisocial and self-defeating traits.'

What did he know? I thought to myself. I had known Larry as well as anyone for several years, and there was no doubt he was like Dad. Indeed, no matter what Judge Camp ruled, it would either tip Larry into depression or, perhaps, provoke a high.

Judge Camp recognised that Larry's untreated 'mental illness' was contributing to the decision to die. 'Mr Lonchar's depression, with its feelings of hopelessness and lack of self-worth, affects his decision-making.' That might be enough for victory. 'Mr Lonchar's decision to forgo further appeals is not one with which most members of society can agree.' Surely this was leading up to the conclusion that no sensible person would follow that course? 'But it is a rational decision,' he concluded, letting the hammer fall heavily on hope. 'Mr Lonchar believes that life is not worth living . . .' Larry was, then, free to die; the state of Georgia was free to shove him into eternity in the electric chair. It was just a matter of time, and throwing the switch.

I was sad and angry in equal measure. The government was a corporate hypocrite.

When Dad had lost all his money, and had no other outlet for his frustrated dreams, he had turned on his family. It had been the worst of times. Now, Larry's sister, Chris Kellogg, bore the brunt of Larry's vitriol. The first time we had asked her to be Larry's 'next friend', she came alone. The second time, her husband was there for support and she had fretted and smoked her way around the filing cabinets every day as we prepared Larry's appeals in her name. Since then she had visited Larry, and sat silently through his cascading complaints. He attacked her bitterly for leaving the family when they were children, for not caring about their mother, or for only appearing on the scene when the newspapers and the lawyers shamed her into it. Larry was not looking for a discussion. He was trying to hurt her, lashing out.

'She never bothered to come and see me for the first two years I was locked up. She's only coming now so she can sleep better when I die. She's just doing this for her guilt. She has stacks of money somewhere,' he said, with no more evidence than her husband's name, Kellogg, mixed with family rumour. 'If only she would come up with fifty grand, I could buy my way out of this and out of prison.'

Larry had known her for a lifetime. The armour of age might protect her from the barbs of strangers, but Larry remembered where the childhood chinks had been, finding them by instinct. Dad did the same with his sister, Auntie Jean, when he labelled her a middle-class woman with a middle-class mind.

'Why did he say these things?' Chris wailed to her husband, confined in their claustrophobic motel room.

Why does the rabid dog bite his owner? Because she is the one who is closest.

Chris's resolve weakened as she listened to Larry's arguments, each of which carried truth. The prison did treat him as an animal. He had no hope of freedom ever again. Because she rarely saw him when he was not trying to get himself killed, to her he seemed unerring in his desire to die. She began to doubt my certainty that Larry would change his mind again if only we stayed with him. She just could not be the 'next friend' any more.

When she fled the field, Larry's antennae turned towards me. I saw him far more than my other clients, because he needed it, yet I was now living in New Orleans. The US is vast, and I was driving 100,000 miles a year. One of the arithmetical sums I had worked out during my endless trips was that if I set my cruise control at 75 mph rather than the ridiculous speed limit (55 mph on the vast highways, engineered for twice that), I would save three forty-hour weeks on the road a year. I had fuzz busters (radar detectors) fore and aft on my car, so I could pinpoint most cops a mile away. I got surprisingly few speeding tickets, but the odd fine was worth it.

A visit to Larry was a round trip of a thousand miles. I could never get there more than once a month, often less frequently. I arrived as soon as I could when Judge Camp delivered his ruling. I began the visit with the normal pleasantries about the recent sports pages. Larry was different today. It seemed as if his eyes were swollen, the corneas bulging towards me. He would not look in my direction. His eyes rolled up towards the top of his skull. He bent his neck, and stared at the ceiling of the visitation room. It was whitewashed concrete, perfect prison polish, with no mark but the imperfections in the final trowelwork. Larry stared intently. He said nothing in reply. It seemed as if the element in the base of the kettle was heating up, gradually boiling up to his mouth.

'Why are you *doin'* this to me?' he said, his voice low. 'Why can't you just *leave me be*?' His venom burst out with a spray of white spittle.

I sat silently, waiting out the storm.

His hands began shaking. His anger rose, along with his voice. I tried to hush him, as if he were a child. 'Larry, we've gotta keep it down or they'll' – a jerk over my shoulder to the door – 'come busting in.' Larry usually responded to being on a team fighting against the prison.

'Why are you *doin'* this?' he said again, his voice louder still. His eyes were manic. He was now pacing.

This time the guard, his chair leaning up against the wall, looked down to see what was happening. Larry heard him move. It made him angry that the prison would intervene, and he lashed out. There was only one person in range. He shoved me. It was no kind of physical threat, though it shocked me. Larry had never come close to being aggressive with me. None of my clients had – least of all him. My mind still told me that I had nothing to worry about.

In a moment, the room was full of uniformed guards. I wanted to get between them and Larry, since I thought they were going to attack him.

'Inmate Lonchar, against the wall!' the officer in charge ordered. He strode forward, gripped my arm and pulled me towards the door.

'Wait . . .' I said, confusion still outweighing any emotion. Above all else, though, I knew I did not want to leave. If I did not talk him down now I might lose him forever.

'Get out of here, now!' The officer's voice was as harsh to me as it had been to Larry.

'But—'

'That's an order. You leave now or you may never come back!' he barked, as two of his guards escorted me out by the shoulder. My instinctive reaction was to tell him he had no power to do this, but I was shoved on my way before I could form the words.

I barely caught a look back over my shoulder. The rest of them did not seem to be putting a hand on Larry, but I was half pushed to the yellow electric gates, and pressed past the ultra-violet scanner without pause.

'You'll have to leave the institution,' another officer told me officiously.

I was calming down. 'I need to see the warden,' I said.

'He's not available,' the officer said. He was clearly just making that up.

'I'll wait,' I said.

In the event, I was led almost directly into Warden Zant's office, where he was almost polite. He seemed to expect me to join the forces of the administration, as though as I was suddenly convinced of the inexorable violence of all inmates. I began to explain that this was Larry's 'mental illness' acting, that he had just had bad news, and that I needed to get back in there to help bring him down. I told him that a doctor does not leave a patient who is sick, and neither should I as his lawyer. Zant listened for a moment before telling me it would be impossible.

'You'll have to leave the institution,' he echoed. 'It's for your own safety.'

My own safety! How could I leave Larry in a moment of anguish like this? But I had to capitulate, and I walked despondently along the subterranean tunnel to the front gate. I was not sure whether I would ever see Larry again. I was vanquished.

Larry was clearly manic; I was depressed. It hurt to work day and night for him only to be told that I was the cause of all his pain. I knew this was not really what he meant, even though there was some truth to it, but Judge Camp had let him down. Larry did not need to be told that he was right to want to die; he needed to hear that he was worth something. But this precipitated a new bout of self-doubt on my part. Was I really just torturing Larry to vindicate my own philosophical goals? Dealing with my own guilt? Could I honestly promise him, or even myself, that I could achieve anything for him?

Three days later, I received a letter from Larry. It was addressed to 'Mr Smith', which was the most hurtful aspect.

It's sad what happened yesterday in the visiting room. They did right by removing you from me. When I was standing and walking it was my way of restraining myself. I'm sure I couldn't have lasted much longer. I went back and called my ex-sister like I informed you I would do. The conversation was very short and painful. Before the end of our conversation she said the lawyers had told her if I signed the appeal papers they could get me a new trial and I'd walk free. Why do you lawyers always lie to get what you all want?

So I had to tell her what I didn't ever want to tell my family, 'Chris, I killed all three of those people. I'm never going free. The lawyers been lying to you to get what they want.' She hung up on me. Her last words to me were, 'I'll call Mr Mears and Mr Smith and inform them not to appeal the judge's ruling. I'm no longer your sister.' (She then hung up.) You all have hurt me and my family very much. Now I've lost my sister 'cause of that and I'll lose some other family members.

I hold you all responsible. I'll have payback (revenge). To avoid this, accept my advice and don't appeal Judge Camp's ruling. If you all do, I promise there will be a 'payback'. Mr Mears has a wife to think of, you are young, don't do it. I have some friends (from Michigan prisons) that one day (you all will have to worry what day) will give me my satisfaction.

He added a postscript: 'I couldn't write this yesterday 'cause I was too upset.'

There was no sign-off 'Sorry!'

I sat at my desk, staring out the window. I didn't buy for a minute that Larry was really confessing to murdering the three people. We knew for sure that Mitch had pulled the trigger. Larry was painting himself further into a corner, to push his family away and help himself through the gates of Hades. I didn't even pause to think about his 'threat' – nobody in Michigan was going to come down to kill me, or Mike. But I did hesitate when it came to appealing Judge Camp's ruling.

Eventually, after morosely studying the wall of the building opposite for a while, I turned to the next thing in my in-tray. The Supreme Court had just issued a ruling in *Stringer* v. *Black*;

my friend Ken Rose had won it for James Stringer based on the vagueness of one of the legal 'aggravating circumstances' where the jury had found the crime to be 'especially heinous, atrocious or cruel'. Since, to the average person, any murder is 'especially atrocious' as compared to any other crime, it was a meaningless way to distinguish between capital crimes, and yet it was meant to justify the death penalty. The Supreme Court ruling was extraordinarily good news, promising a new sentencing trial for a number of people on Mississippi's death row. As I read the opinion, I remembered that it was the very issue that we had raised, and lost, for Edward Johnson five years before. Indeed, the 'Death Squad' Assistant Attorney General, Sonny White, had argued to the Supreme Court justices in Washington that the ruling in *Johnson* v. *Thigpen* dictated that Stringer should lose.

'The short answer to the state's argument,' the court now wrote, 'is that the Fifth Circuit made a serious mistake in *Johnson* v. *Thigpen*. Use of a vague or imprecise aggravating factor in the weighing process invalidates the sentence.'

Edward, they said, should never have been executed. But his body had long been buried in the Walnut Grove graveyard.

25

A Juror's Betrayal

Midway through life's journey
I found myself in a dark wood . . .
I cannot well recall how I entered there
So full of sleep was I when
I lost my way.

Dante, Inferno, Canto 1

Brian Jardine's house was in an expensive suburb. It was shuttered from peering eyes, with a double garage off to the right. A ginger cat watched my approach with minimal interest. There was a sense of oppression – part the Georgia humidity, part a feeling of being watched from the other houses. The alarm systems were not the true deterrent: it had taken me an hour just to find the street. When I stopped at the fire station to ask for directions, a friendly member of the emergency response team had taken twenty minutes to find the street on his map. The whole place would be ashes long before the red fire truck wailed into the cul-de-sac.

I knocked on the front door. I was nervous. I had driven the five hundred miles from New Orleans on a whim, thinking it was time I spoke to the jurors. There was no guarantee that anyone would want to talk to me. The only black woman who had been on Larry's jury had refused earlier that afternoon. Juror No. 3, Brian Jardine, had been the only white man, and he had voted that Larry should die. I heard someone shuffling around. I sensed an eye being pressed against the peephole, so I tried to look friendly and keep my hands in plain view. The bolt slid back. A diffident, grey-haired man peered around the door. I began to explain why I was there.

He said he would have to check with his wife whether she minded him talking to me tonight. It was eight o'clock and getting dark. His head slid back around the door, leaving it ajar as he disappeared into the house. Part of me wanted to go to my hotel room and watch a bad film. Part of me did not want to talk to anyone who had voted for Larry's death. Brian came back quickly, pulling the door open.

'I can talk for fifteen minutes,' he conceded, 'seeing you've come all this way.' He offered me the chair to the left of the front door, barely into the sitting room, my left arm leaning against an expensive desk, where an open leather-bound book and glasses suggested he had just been reading. I knew that Brian was a sales associate, and this was his Friday-evening relaxation. He sat down, clearly tense in his pastel-striped shirt and green shorts. He had kicked off his shoes. As he spoke, it became clear that his life was regimented rather than contemplated. When he took off his other glasses, large and oval, he looked vulnerable, the clear lines of his world blurred.

I began with generalities about the trial, jotting surreptitious notes down on a pad that I would type up later that evening. Brian soon warmed to his subject, and described what it was like to be asked to decide whether a fellow human should die. 'They took the books off the other jurors,' he remembered. 'Then the bailiff, she saw what I was reading. It was the *US Sales Annual.* "Guess you can keep that," she said to me. "Can't have anything in there about the case."'

How did being a sales associate give him any training to handle the question of whether Larry should die?

'I kinda resented the approach the court had with the jurors. They'd throw you in a room, wouldn't give you any help, just leave you there.' Brian spoke with vehemence.

His wife, Barbara, appeared. She was small, with a round face and a wan complexion. While she was initially less open than her husband, she gradually took over the conversation. I imagined the same had happened in their marriage.

In addition to Brian, the lone white man, and the one black woman, there were five white women and five black men on Larry's jury – balanced, in a state where black people are routinely excluded from jury service. 'We deliberated for two and a half days. Started on a Thursday, went all day Friday, and into Saturday. We had to agree. I think the judge told us that, but I don't remember now. But we felt we had to agree. So we just talked it over from every angle.'

I explained to him that the jurors had misunderstood. They did not have to agree. They could have agreed to disagree within five minutes of starting their discussion and Larry would have lived. This did not seem to register. It gradually became clear that Brian had not been one of the jurors with any doubts.

'To begin with, I think the five black men were for life,' he said. He paused, as if he wondered whether he was about to say something he should not. 'I guess they were more used to violent stuff. We talked about what it would mean if we gave him life. I remember there was violent opposition to life from the white ladies. They felt like he would get out and probably do the same thing again.'

Brian had no doubt that Larry had committed the crime, just as the prosecution said he did.

'It was a slam-dunk,' he said resolutely, then, uncertain whether a sporting analogy was appropriate, added hesitatingly: '. . . if I may use that expression?' Then his tone became firm again. 'It was execution-style. They put cuffs on two of them, then shot them execution-style. And he came back and stabbed the woman too.'

Did he think that perhaps Larry was suicidal, anticipating that the electric chair might one day bring him relief?

'No, we thought he was just bad, a killer,' Brian said emphatically. 'He was very intimidating . . . he had wild looks in his eyes.' That interested me. Larry did get wild eyes, but only when he was manic. 'We did an earnest, sincere job. I don't know what else we could have done. We asked ourselves, "Can we really give him life?" Life means he's paroled, and he'll kill again. We just looked at him as a killer.' Brian's diction was very precise.

When I told him that Larry was manic-depressive, and that I had spent several years preventing him from ending his own life, Brian was quiet. I could feel that Barbara, too, was tense. I was tempted to interrupt the silence, as a long pause can remind a person you're interviewing that it is time for you to leave. But as the stillness crescendoed, I knew that I had imparted some terrible truth.

'We're mental health advocates,' Brian blurted finally. There was a small, unpleasant part of me that was pleased to see his discomfort, given that he had voted for Larry's death. It was churlish, and it had not been my purpose to come into their home to make Brian feel guilty.

'I feel betrayed,' he said, in obvious pain. 'I feel like I should have known that. You can't execute someone who's mentally ill.'

I wondered aloud what had turned them into such committed 'advocates'. I mentioned my father, and said – sincerely – how much I appreciated what they were doing. Brian looked at his wife. She did not even glance back.

'Our son,' she began, 'Kurt . . . they say he's schizophrenic – but then they used to say he's manic-depressive. I'm not sure that there's always much difference. He had his first "episode" when he started high school.'

'He thought he had bugs on him,' Brian said. 'I lay down with him and held him to me, to try to tell him that there weren't any bugs.' He announced it so rationally, as if Kurt should have believed him. I was not sure how far I could explore the tragedy of their son, but once Barbara had started, she was not going to be stopped.

'Is it real? I still ask myself that,' she said, confusion still fresh after several years. 'Of course, it was a while before we worked out what was really wrong. The first time, he had to go away. He hated us for that. We would try to have him at home, but there was no structure. We would keep him locked in his room. Maybe it was the opposite of what he needed, but that was the advice we got at the time.

'When there is a crisis in the family, he gets into his episodes. He gets loopy,' Barbara continued. I was taken aback by the word. 'That was before his medication, of course. And when Brian was on the jury, I thought it was going to happen again. But it wasn't so bad that time, he didn't really go off.'

They had decided to take choice away from him. 'We've become guardians for our son,' Brian said. 'Now we can force him to take his medication, we can commit him, like that.' He snapped his fingers.

'A mentally ill person should not be allowed to refuse medicine,' Barbara added. 'Kurt may know right from wrong, but he's not rational. Sometimes he just doesn't know what he's done. He chased me with a knife once. He's strong. Our oldest son was here, and he's got training, been in the navy. He took it off him. Kurt's never mentioned it. I don't think he knows he did it.'

I mentioned that Larry still did not believe he had attacked his mother. Both nodded knowingly.

'No, Kurt doesn't make rational decisions,' Brian said firmly.

I asked, tentatively, whether Kurt had ever tried to kill himself. In the chaotic world that whirled around their son, this was apparently a normal question: three times, or was it four? 'They blur together. She's the one with the elephant memory,' Brian said, looking at Barbara fondly.

'The first time he overdosed on medications,' said Barbara, counting them off matter-of-factly. 'I heard him throwing up. He had taken fifty pills. You know the charcoal treatment? They give you liquid charcoal to absorb the pills. It's a horrible treatment.'

'I thought he'd learned never to do it again,' Brian said.

Kurt tried the drug route twice more.

'We dropped him off at the hospital, the last time,' said Brian. 'We told them, when the charcoal treatment's finished, just take him upstairs to the psych ward. Just take him right on up there.'

'If we hadn't taken care of him, he'd be either dead or on the street,' said Barbara. She paused. She seemed to be looking inward as she went on talking. 'He'd probably be dead of his own hand. If I was mentally ill I don't know that I wouldn't want to be dead. He's bright, and was so musical. And I think he's depressed because he's getting older, and has nothing to look forward to.'

For some reason it seemed acceptable to ask them what they thought about taking their own lives.

'I've thought about suicide,' Barbara replied calmly, as if she were considering retirement. 'I've had heart trouble, other things. My friend is a counsellor, she talked to me. She accused me of thinking about suicide, that I was choosing not to live as a way out of my problems . . . not so much the illnesses, as Kurt. It has been an immense loss, losing my son.'

Kurt was almost a character from Christmas Past, a relative like my great-grandmother Frances Canham, who had been dropped off at the Fulbourn Asylum in 1912. The futility of Barbara's life draped around her, heavy even in the air conditioning of their home. 'I guess for a while I couldn't choose to get over my illness. I could choose not to get over it. I knew I needed to get on, but it's the guilt. It's like an old dog that buries a bone and keeps on going back to dig it up.'

I explained how I had come to take on Larry's case. I wondered what duty – or what right – they thought I might have to stop Larry from killing himself.

'You've no right to stop him,' Barbara said. She was certain that suicide was a rational decision, not just for the terminally ill. 'He should be allowed to make the final decision. In Larry's shoes, I would not want to live.'

'It may be a rational decision, and I might even opt for it,' Brian began. 'But I don't think it should be allowed. I don't think we can afford to let people be killing themselves in prison. There has to be a certain order. You get a death sentence, then you have to be executed. You get a life sentence, then you have to pay for it. You can't let people be just taking their own lives in prison.' He paused. Disorder had obviously entered his ordered world in the shape of Kurt, and it was now rearing back in the form of Larry. 'No. Even out of prison, if there was any way to prevent it, I would stop it.'

So how did Brian feel about being put in the position of voting to give Larry what he apparently wanted?

'I don't feel like I am an accomplice to his suicide,' he initially said, sure of himself. 'Or maybe I do, in a bizarre way.' He was silent for what seemed like a long time. 'I'm disgusted that we didn't get that information. If it's the defendant's right to veto presenting evidence of "mental illness", I don't think that's right. He can't make that decision. If Larry wanted the death penalty, I'd say he was mentally ill and he wasn't entitled to make that call. I feel betrayed.'

I had been invited in for fifteen minutes, which had now run into four hours. It was almost midnight. We had none of us moved in that time, not even for the statutory Southern glass of iced tea. I thanked them for their time. I noticed that Brian had never mentioned Larry's last name. He was Larry to Brian, as he was to me.

26

Dad Writes Poetry to Five-Year-Old Girls

> We'll turn the darkness into Light!
> We'll tame the Devil if we can. . .
>
> Dad, 'Ode to Mistress Silke'

In the mid-1990s Dad was approaching seventy, and the changes were becoming more obvious. We had found him a two-room flat in the centre of the small city of Ely, just next to a residential home to which perhaps he would graduate one day not too far off. It was a midnight in October. Dad had been up much of the night, and had completed a poem to the daughter of some neighbours, a young girl called Silke. There were those who whispered when an old, stooped man started sending poems to a five-year-old girl, but apparently that thought never crossed his mind. He dedicated the ode to Mistress Silke and sent a copy to the *Telegraph*.

> The days are dark, the spirit's cold –
> The lamps burn low, and hearts beat slow.
> The hounds of Hell are baying bold
> And all the world awaits the blow,
> The fall of Fate. What will it be?
> The comet's crash? A plague that kills?
> The H-bomb's blast? And shall we see
> Our Spirit break before these ills?
> Or will the long-evolving Man
> End in disaster and defeat?
> Will all God's dreams since Life began

Revert to ashes at His feet?
No! No! Our Spirit shall not fail
As long as you are here to fight;
To struggle on to tell the tale
And see the dawn transcend the night!
We'll turn the darkness into Light!
We'll tame the Devil if we can,
And then we'll strive with all our might
To work towards our perfect plan!

There was nothing nefarious about it. Dad enthused kids, whose company he often preferred to the adults who had long since been tainted by conformity. And by now, he had driven most of his adult friends away.

When I came across this poem, I thought it quite good. I have edited it slightly – taking out as many references to 'Man' as I could (half a dozen), and making a few other minor word changes. That I am doing it now only illustrates how late I am in coming to the party. If I had done that when he wrote it, he would have been delighted; it would have been an interaction where we could have forged a true alliance.

Not for the first time, I wondered the extent to which Dad could have been steered away from his periodic rampages if someone like me – with both an interest and an obligation – had spent a little of the time I devoted to my clients pressing on the positive elements of his personality, rather than simply trying to keep him at bay.

We have different options when we deal with the varied temperaments of those whose lives touch our own: we can struggle against them, or we can try to identify the passions that drive them, and what can reasonably work for them. Dad could not create a business and run it with any chance of success – that much was clear. He could, perhaps, have ideas that he might pass on to someone with a talent for implementation. Dad should be kept as far away as possible from the various forms of gambling, or any get-rich-quick notion.

Vincent van Gogh cut his ear off and ultimately took his own life, but when he was painting he had a channel that was well suited to his energies and interfered with nobody else. The obvious avenue for Dad was poetry. Like anyone, Dad needed appreciation. Society does not readily pay people to potter around in their poetry sheds, but it would have been less expensive, and taken much less energy, to underwrite him with this passion than to try to squeeze him into one of the professions advocated fifty years before by his school. In any event, by now Dad had a pension and was free to spend all of his time on poetry – but someone had to encourage him.

As a family, we might have found Dad incorrigible, but in retrospect his life could have been salvaged. As a society, we have some foolish responses to those we don't understand. This is well illustrated by some of the most unpopular people I have ever represented, people who are hated far more even than Larry: paedophiles.

If the *Telegraph* had published Dad's claim that he was "'Neath the window of Five-Year-Old Mistress Silke next the Moonlit River Ouse', the paedophile vigilantes would have flooded the low-lying city of Ely. Indeed, at that time a wave of hysteria had just swept the country after the *News of the World* started to publish lists of convicted sex offenders. In August 2000, paediatric specialist Dr Yvette Cloete would be run out of her home in the small South Wales village of St Brides, when some locals who could not comprehend her professional title daubed the word 'paedo' on her cottage.

Defending Ricky Langley probably taught me more about the problem than anything else. He was so notorious that Louisiana enacted a Scarlet Letter law where convicted sex offenders had to send postcards to all their neighbours when they moved into a new home. My wife and I received two such missives in New Orleans while we lived there. We went round to the address to offer help if the person faced harassment, but the bricks had already been hurled through the windows, the transient tenant run out of town. Thus, someone who very likely suffered with a serious disorder was driven underground, and would probably end up harming someone else.

Ricky's story began in 1963, before he was conceived. His father, Alcide, drunk, was driving along in their old car, wife Bessie in the passenger seat, and two kids without seat belts in the back. Alcide drove into a telegraph pole. Both kids were killed. One, Oscar Lee, a tousle-haired six-year-old, had been the apple of Alcide's eye. Bessie went through the front window and was in Charity Hospital, in a body cast, for much of the next two years. At some point during her confinement, Alcide insisted on his conjugal rights, and Bessie conceived Ricky James Langley. Nobody believed her when she said she thought she was pregnant. At five months they finally cut off the cast and – whoosh! – her belly expanded.

The doctors told her she must have an abortion. The foetus had been through countless X-rays, in addition to many medical toxins. Alcide, though, said that as a Catholic he could not countenance abortion. Thus, the child was born, a fact that Ricky always regretted. He was exposed *in utero* to one drug, we discovered, that has been linked to subsequent paedophilia, though I did not think anyone would believe it so we did not present this to Ricky's jury – they would have thought we made it up.

Ricky was never going to be a replacement for the blond Oscar Lee. He had Coke-bottle glasses, and greasy brown hair that failed to disguise his protuberant ears. By seven, he was being sexually molested by a cousin. He began sleeping on gravestones, and at eleven he posted a note on the school board – 'I am not Ricky Langley, I am Oscar Lee Langley.' The prosecution later suggested that he was preparing for an insanity defence . . .

Though he knew he was 'different', he had no idea what that difference was when he was first arrested, in Georgia, for molesting a young girl. He was sent to prison where, for the first time, a therapist identified his 'mental illness', and told him that he was incurable and he would inevitably reoffend. Over many years, Ricky impressed me with his intelligence. Even though he inhabited a distinct universe to mine, he could see the clear consequences of his diagnosis: he did not want to go out into everyone else's world and harm a child. Therefore he demanded – fortunately, in writing – that the Georgia State Board of Pardons and Paroles not release him. He was ignored, and sent back to Louisiana on parole. Sure enough, it was a year later that he strangled six-year-old Jeremy Guillory.

I got two chances to keep Ricky from the execution chamber, for which I am deeply grateful. At the first trial we presented a strong insanity defence, and the jury not only convicted him but imposed a death sentence. Later, when we interviewed them, the jurors said they had found our case convincing, and because he was insane they needed to kill Ricky to make sure he did not escape prison and kill again. Though I had failed him the first time around, his conviction was reversed. There were plenty of more substantial reasons why he should have had a new trial, but his conviction was tossed out on an extraordinarily technical issue – he, as a white male, had been indicted by a grand jury (which would proverbially indict a ham sandwich) where the role of foreperson was filled by a white male, excluding minorities and women. Prior to the second trial, I had a better comprehension of the swirling entropy of Ricky's mind, and I had also learned more about the thought process of jurors in those ten extra years.

I also spent time with Lorilei Guillory – Jeremy's mother. Lorilei would rightly say that it is not my place to speak for her, but I think she wanted to understand why her treasure had been ripped from her, and to obtain some reassurance that his final moments had not been as ghastly as she feared. The prosecution, intent on securing death for Ricky, had suggested – falsely – that Ricky had sexually molested Jeremy. I don't think he had. Ricky explained to me in strangely rational tones that when Jeremy came to the door of his apartment, he recognised Oscar Lee, whom he saw as his very real dead brother who made him want to molest children.

'Can I meet Oscar Lee?' I asked him at one of our many meetings.

'I don't see why not. S'long as he wants to meet you.' Intellectually, he knew that I, along with everyone but himself, thought Oscar Lee did not actually exist. Oscar Lee existed for him.

Lorilei made many brave decisions; one was that she wanted to meet with Ricky, who she had always referred to as 'Langley'. I arranged for her to spend three hours with him at the Calcasieu Parish Jail. Retrospectively, he knew now what he had done. He knew the pain he had caused. He wanted to apologise and explain as best he could to this mother, who was still grieving ten years on, and would be for the rest of her life.

'Ricky,' she said after three hours talking to him, shifting to his Christian name, 'I'm going to fight for you.' And fight she did. When she announced that she wanted no revenge, the district attorney tried to have her declared an unfit mother, so he could take away her second child. She taught me many things, and one was an important distinction: she was never, she thought, going to forgive Ricky for what he had done, but she did want to show mercy. Ultimately, while she testified for the prosecution to tell the jury what she knew of the dreadful day Jeremy went missing, she insisted on coming back to the witness stand for the defence. She instructed me on the only question she wanted to answer.

'Ms Guillory,' I asked, 'from your interactions with Ricky Langley, do you have an opinion as to his mental state?'

'Yes, as a matter of fact, I do,' she replied firmly. She turned to the twelve jurors, all of whom understood this to be the moment of highest human drama. She managed to pierce even my carapace, and get me weeping. 'In my opinion . . . I feel like Ricky Langley has cried out for help many, many, many times. And for whatever reason, his family, society, and the system has failed him. I feel like he is sick . . . And even though, as I sit on this witness stand, I can hear my child's death cry' – her voice trembled – 'I can hear Ricky Langley cry for help too. And for whatever reason, he has never gotten the help he needed . . . in my opinion.' She made it clear that he should be in a psychiatric hospital not a prison, although she also wanted to be clear that he should never be released.

The aptly named Cynthia Killingsworth, prosecuting, tried to undermine her, pointing out that Lorilei had met Ricky only twice. This ignored the essence of what this devastated mother had to say: she was struggling to go beyond condemnation. It was the shortest closing argument I ever had to give in a death penalty case. Lorilei remains to this day one of my heroes. She was able to peer through the gloom to see what led Ricky to do what he had done. She might never forgive him. She might often want him dead. But she was still able to show the compassion that the government – the omnipotent teacher, for good and for ill – would have her refuse.

Ricky is still alive today, thanks to Lorilei.

We had a panel of twelve good jurors, all of whom had personal exposure to people close to them with 'mental disorders'. They respected Lorilei – as they told me later, when two of them became my friends – and they acquitted him of capital murder. Both Lorilei and Ricky wanted him in a psychiatric hospital forever, but the prosecution had lied to the jury, saying he would be released if found not guilty by reason of insanity. The jurors therefore voted him guilty of a lesser offence, so he would remain in prison. For this reason, the verdict was reversed yet again, and Lorilei would have to endure another two trials.

The fact of Ricky's paedophilia highlights our own limits of understanding. Every expert who evaluated Ricky said he was incurable. Meanwhile, nobody hates Ricky more than Ricky himself. When I give talks that touch on this topic, and am confronted by a hateful rant, I always ask the crowd: who would choose to be a paedophile? Normally, there is a nervous titter.

Paedophilia is our twenty-first-century leprosy. Until the 1940s, we had little understanding and no cure for the leper. They were kept in colonies, and the very word became a synonym for 'outcast'. Our ministers of religion taught us to spurn them, and blame them for their own illness. 'He is a leprous man, he is unclean: the priest shall pronounce him utterly unclean; his plague is in his head. And the leper . . . shall cry, Unclean, unclean. All the days wherein the plague shall be in him he shall be defiled; he is unclean: he shall dwell alone; without the camp shall his habitation be' (Leviticus 13: 44–46).

Paedophiles are likewise condemned through our ignorance: it is barbaric to blame Ricky Langley for the fact that we have no cure. Ricky would be the first person to say that he needs to be quarantined – indeed he wrote to the Georgia parole board to demand that he not be released – but we need to approach this as we would someone suffering from a contagious disease. He is a victim. We needed to recognise this before he killed Jeremy Guillory, instead of passing Scarlet Letter laws.

I have made a habit of defending paedophiles, because it is the natural extension of what my mother taught me – that life is all about helping people who are worse off than we are. There is nobody whom we hate more than paedophiles. However, Ricky Langley illustrates our own failings far more clearly than even my father did. For now, we have no solution to offer him.

27

Suicide by Electric Chair

When the executioner throws the switch that sends the electric current through the body, the prisoner cringes from torture, his flesh swells and his skin stretches to the point of breaking.

William J. Brennan Jr, Justice of the US Supreme Court

Larry was hardly likely to be hiring hit men to assassinate Mike Mears and me. However, the FBI called Mike to say that they had intercepted a letter to one of Larry's old friends in jail up north, soon to be released, asking for a favour – to carry out his threat for old times' sake.

Mike and I met for a drink at the Station, a bar in Decatur where he was still greeted as 'Mr Mayor'. Neither of us took the threat seriously: the letter had never been delivered, and Mike had already told the feds not to follow it up. It was just a poker game for Larry. He knew his letters were censored, and he would have used code – he often had with me – if he wanted a real message to get through. The fact that he did not suggested that he expected the letter to be intercepted, and that we would be told. We agreed, though, that if we made light of his Michigan Mafia, it would aggravate him. He needed us to believe in the mirage of convict life, where the bond between convicts was so strong that someone who had finally received his freedom would risk it all to kill for a fellow con.

Contrary to his wishes, we did file the appeal, but I went as supplicant to Larry to ask him to call off his dogs. He strung me along for the first visit with an endless litany of examples of the barbaric way that he was being treated at the 'Diagnostic

Center': the guards were calling him Loony Larry, the summer thermometer was rising, and his family had deserted him once again. Still, with volunteer students coming in over the summer months, Larry got visits on a weekly basis to cheer him up. Eventually, he officially withdrew the threats, returning to his amiable, albeit self–destructive, self. While I was pleased to be back in Larry's favour, we were getting no closer to persuading him back on board. The federal appellate court would soon rule, probably allowing Larry to die. Then the Supreme Court would be the only barrier between him and oblivion. The state would have its pound of flesh.

It was noon on Ash Wednesday 1995, in a state with the electric chair. Larry would die in just seven hours. We had asked the Board of Pardons for a ninety-day stay so that the prison could be required to medicate Larry. The previous night the board said that no hearing would be necessary; the inevitable word 'DENIED' had come this morning. No lithium pill would cure what they had planned for him today.

All week I had been in court on behalf of Emmanuel Hammond. Emmanuel wanted to live, though most of Georgia wanted him to die – a black man from the projects who had allegedly raped and killed Julie Love, an innocent white woman. In the media, he had been portrayed as a hulking personification of evil, but the angle of their cameras dictated perceptions. He was a skinny five foot nine, his face pockmarked from a bad case of childhood acne. Mike Mears had asked me to help when he took on the case, payback for Larry. At least this time we had one person – Emmanuel – on our side.

I was getting ready to head out of the courtroom shortly after lunchtime, leaving Mike to continue alone. I had to get down to the prison for the execution. One of the police bailiffs pulled me aside.

'You representing that Lonchar guy?' he demanded. I pulled back a little from his hand, knowing what to expect from this white man with a crew cut and a uniform: *the sonofabitch wants to die . . . he deserves to die . . . why won't you let him die?*

'Good luck,' the man said softly, checking that none of his superiors were in earshot. 'What they're doing to him just ain't right. I hope you can stop it.'

I have no idea what I said. I hope I thanked him properly.

All week Mike and I had waged war against the two prosecutors who were trying to ensure Emmanuel's execution. I prefer a prosecutor who is a short, scarred fascist with a supercilious attitude; at least you know he was abused in the playground. Emmanuel's prosecutors did not fit my stereotype. They came up to me as I was stuffing papers in the battered black briefcase I had kept since law school. 'Good luck tonight,' each said in turn.

One had been a public defender. 'The pay's better on this side,' he had told me when I asked why he switched. 'And you don't have to stay up all night when they kill your clients. I would not be back on the defence side for anything. I just can't imagine having to go down there when they are going to kill one of my clients.' It was strange to think of a hired gun, able to take either side of Life and Death.

There was a parking ticket on the car when I got to it. It was raining. I had hoped it was cold enough to risk an extra half an hour on the meter. I had gambled and lost. It was going to be that kind of evening. A ten-dollar fine now; Larry's life later.

When I arrived at the prison, Larry announced that he had decided not to tell me the numbers he had been playing on the lotto for the past five years. 'I've told my mom to carry on playing them. I know I'm goin' to hell, you know . . .' His voice was despondent, distilled. For someone who insisted that he could not believe in God, Larry had no doubt about eternal damnation. 'But maybe there'll be time . . . maybe I'll have a little time before I go there. Maybe I'll be able to work the numbers. If there's anything I can do to manipulate the result, I don't want any split tickets. I don't want her to share with you or nobody. I want her to get it all. Least I can do, after all I've let her down.'

There was a small part of me that, against all the odds, felt slightly aggrieved that the charity I was working for would not benefit at all from the massive win – Powerball was into the hundreds of millions.

Now it was after 3 p.m. Warden Zant had told me that Larry's family had to leave the prison in half an hour. Larry was deeply depressed, but on the surface he seemed ready to die. I explained to him that I would be there, in the prison and in the witness room, right up to the moment that they killed him. I did not mean to sound harsh, but there was no way to describe it kindly. I was caught between needing to break through the unreality of the moment, yet not wanting to destroy the dignity that he was trying to hold together. He listened; he nodded. No more. He went back to chatting with his father and his brother. At the best of times, both were the type who would say nothing at the dinner table on Thanksgiving. They were confused and embarrassed by having to come up with something to discuss for half an hour before losing the son and brother they had never really talked to.

I was struggling to think of a way to get through to him, with the time ebbing away. Larry still did not seem to view the upcoming execution as his own. He was speaking in the third person, as if he were a spectator. I decided I had to focus him on death, so that he might realise it was worth avoiding before it was too late.

'What did you do about your Last Statement, Larry?' I asked.

'I worked on it, but it isn't right. It's not what I want to say.' He pulled a piece of paper out of his pocket. 'I want to die,' Larry had written. 'I have written down this Statement because I am so scared that I can't speak. I wish I could live my life over again and make my parents proud, but I can't do that. Maybe death will be better than my life. Who knows? When I was a little boy I was, in a way, an all-American kid,' he lied, rewriting history for the sake of his family. 'I played Little League, had a newspaper route, and was a Cub Scout. But things went sour. I felt guilty. I felt that I had somehow caused my parents' separation. I've hated myself ever since.'

The cynical public believes that everyone on death row gets religion as death approaches. Larry had even missed out on this luxury.

I go to my death without a belief in God. I've wanted to believe very hard, but just haven't been able to. I've prayed, but nothing has happened. I'll continue to pray when I'm strapped in the chair. I hope with all my heart that there is somewhere a God who loves me. One thing that confuses me a lot is the way so many Christians think about the death penalty. In the Sermon on the Mount, Jesus preaches forgiveness. His whole life down to his death on the Cross was about forgiving others. It must have really taken something for him to have forgiven those Roman soldiers at the foot of the Cross. I wish I had that kind of faith.

I want to say to my family how much I owe them. My mother, especially, has been so good and faithful to me, even though I've let her and the whole family down all the years I've been in prison. This tears me apart – I love all my family more than they'll ever know. If there is a God, may this God watch over them all. May God watch over this whole planet.

And that was it. The poor player who struts and frets his last hour upon the stage. The warden would signal to the executioner, the electric chair would soon start to buzz.

His handwriting was impeccable, no shaking had betrayed him. He was simply not writing about *his* death. It was a work of fiction. In front of me, in the visiting room, Larry was talking about another person. He was floating, his eyes on the ceiling once again, detached from the surreal world around him. At that moment, I was convinced that he was out of touch with reality under any sensible definition. I refused to say good-bye. I was going to be allowed back in ninety minutes, to spend the last couple of hours within feet of Larry, even if the prison would not let me be in the same room as him. I went out into the hall to leave his father and Chooch to spend their last few minutes with him.

Convinced that he was dissociating, I wondered whether to file a last-minute affidavit about his mental state. But I did not have the courage to fight Larry once again. There was no chance now that he would change his mind. He really was going to die. I paced around. I tried to think of something to say to help the fragments of his family through this, the stran-gest of times. Finally, tired of inaction, I demanded to be let back into the cell where Larry was beginning to say goodbye. His father was a proud man. He probably had not cried in forty years, but he was crying now.

I pulled Larry by the arm to the other end of the long yellow visitation room.

'Do you know what's happening?' I asked. 'We've only got three more hours. You can't let them do this, Larry.'

'Take my dad out of here, man,' he said. He was crying too, now. 'I can't see him like this. It's torture. Take him out of here!'

'I'll do it, Larry. But don't go through with this. It's torture on your dad, too.' Larry tried not to look me in the eye, but I made him do it. 'You know all you have to do. It'll be tough on you, Larry, but you know, and we know, it'll be the braver and harder thing to do now. Do it. Please. Not for me. For your dad. For Chooch, your brother. For your mother.'

I put an arm about Larry's father, and took him out. He was in his early sixties, but the alcohol had left him looking fifteen years older. He had been alone for years, with nobody to help him understand his own life. His daughter had fled to Florida as soon as she could and his three sons had not turned out well:

one an alcoholic, one in and out of prison for drugs, and the third in front of him about to die for murder. People were staring at the old man's tears, so I steered him into the men's room, in the corner beside the junk-food vending machines.

'What did I do?' he pleaded into his handkerchief, sobbing. 'I been looking after my granddaughter . . . she's doin' OK. Maybe I weren't no good as a dad . . . but I did best as I could.' What could I say? A lifetime's guilt cannot be washed away by a few platitudes in a prison toilet. Silence, and a firm grip on his shoulder, eventually calmed him. As soon as I dared, I led him back out into the hall. The prison timetable would not pause long for a parent's grief, and his emotions might not withstand a guard ordering him out.

I had felt this strange stillness before – in Mississippi, as the family left Edward Johnson for the last time. Now my wandering thoughts were disturbed as Chooch came out of the visiting room. Everyone stood there, waiting for Larry to pass by – for one last look. Then a guard came into the hall and said that Larry wanted everyone out of the way before he would leave the visiting room. He had to protect himself from the sense that people cared for him.

We began to walk out. Those final hours were always the hardest for everyone, but for Larry most of all. I was going to try to persuade the warden to let me be there with him. I doubted he would agree, but Don Cabana, the warden at Parchman, had let me stay with Edward right through to the gas chamber. I was no security risk.

Why would they be afraid to have me present? I knew the reason, of course: they did not want me talking him out of dying. At the same time, I did not trust the guards who would be with him: they had to volunteer to be on the execution squad, and what kind of person would do that? If Larry started wavering in his determination to die, they would accuse him of losing his nerve, of cowardice, and try to steel him for his own death.

Warden Walter Zant was a small man, harsh. I did not like

him, but he was not the worst. That title surely went to his equally diminutive deputy, Assistant Warden Willis Marable, who was standing next to him. Some people in prison just 'do their job'; some can be kind in the moment of need; a small number relish their role as the Marquis de Sade. Marable wanted Larry dead.

Neither of them was in the mood to be helpful. 'When you come back in, you come as a witness to the execution,' said the warden. 'There will be no personal access.'

'You're not even his lawyer now,' added Marable, putting as much spleen into his voice as he could manage. 'He doesn't have a lawyer, so you don't have any right to talk to him.'

I would like to have shouted at them. I had been Larry's lawyer all along, just not always doing what he said he wanted. But my mission was not served by being bombastic, so I tried to reason with them. After some back and forth, Zant said I would be allowed to talk to Larry on the phone from inside the prison at 6.15 p.m., forty-five minutes before the execution. It was not enough.

I tried another ploy. 'What happens if there is some legal crisis and I need to talk to him after that?'

'What legal crisis?' demanded Marable aggressively.

Merely having to put up with Marable was a legal crisis. I was about to tell him that it was none of his goddamned business what legal crisis might arise, but Zant was marginally more reasonable. 'If there is some legal reason that a lawyer has to talk to the inmate then we will put a call through,' he said. 'I can't see how it would be you, though, since you will be here in the institution.'

I silenced myself. I already had an idea, and there was no need to tell them about it. I left the prison.

Larry's family were lost-looking, standing outside in the parking lot, an unfriendly place in the shadow of the guard tower. I pretended this was an everyday event, and marched up with the announcement that I had a plan.

'Don't get so down,' I said, with feigned cheer. 'Of course it's not over. We've been much, much closer than this before, and pulled it out. There's over three hours yet.'

It is true an execution may be stayed at the last minute. Most are not. When they are, it is always when the client asks for a stay. And had I been honest, I would have had to admit that I personally had never had a client come this close and not die. I knew it was over, but hope was their opiate.

I strode to my car and drove to the truck-stop diner by the interstate, where I found Larry's other friends hiding their impotence behind the sports pages of the *Atlanta Constitution*. After asking for a cup of the dubious coffee, I began to simulate action as well, calling Mike Mears in Atlanta to have him negotiate directly with the commissioner of the Department of Corrections over access to Larry.

I then outlined the plan of campaign – it sounded optimistic, but to the discerning ear it would grind to a halt when Larry refused to let us file his appeals. The whole focus now had to be on getting as much access to Larry as possible, to try to change his mind.

'Zant told me that he would allow access from the outside, not from me, for any legal emergency,' I said. 'I am going to talk to him at about six fifteen p.m. You allow ten minutes for my call. I want you to call him around six thirty p.m.'

'What should we say we want to talk to him about?' asked Steve Bayliss, another lawyer who had been a good friend to Larry.

'You don't,' I said, since I could not think of anything terribly convincing. 'Tell them you're a lawyer and it's privileged. Only if you can't get away with that, then tell 'em you have an emergency, you need to talk to him about what we filed in Butts County.' That was plausible enough, since we had filed some papers in the local court that afternoon in an effort to leave room for hope. We had come up with a byzantine point of civil procedure that might confuse the Attorney General for a few hours, so that Larry's family had some piece of forensic flotsam to cling on to – for us, writing it up late the night before had been an alternative to paralysis.

'Now, we need to keep some open phone lines from the prison to here,' I said. Selfishly, I did not want to be cut off in there, unable to call a friendly voice. It was going to be lonely in the prison, waiting for them to kill Larry. I wrote down the numbers for the phone at the booth at the diner, for the diner itself, and for the stocky mobile Steve had. 'The moment I get in the prison, I'll call you with a direct number where you can get me.' There was a payphone in the waiting area. A flutter ran down my spine as I remembered that they would not let me take in coins, or even the cards in my wallet. I might have arrived at that final hour armed with contacts for my friends but unable to make a call: the fatal mundane. I copied the number of a telephone credit card, my lifeline.

'Where's Larry's father and Chooch?' Mary Eastland asked. She was a volunteer with the office, sitting at the next table with Murphy Davis and Ed Loring, a married brace of ministers who ran a homeless shelter in Atlanta and had stood solid by every prisoner on death row for a decade. The same powerless faces appeared every time an execution came up.

'Probably at the Hope House,' Murphy said, referring to the trailer home, cobbled together with charitable donations, where families could stay when they were visiting their relatives on death row.

For some reason, I remembered the rules there. 'I thought they didn't allow alcohol at the Hope House. You know, it might be a good idea to make sure Larry's dad has a few beers to help him through this.' He was an alcoholic, and here I was suggesting we give him liquor.

'Oh, I think they allow it, they just don't provide it,' Murphy said with a smile. She obviously agreed that it would be a good idea to anaesthetise Milan.

My back was killing me. I had done something horrible to

myself trying to move a millstone in my garden. I went to the men's room to adjust the ridiculous girdle that the chiropractor had told me to wear, wondering if the prison would think I was trying to smuggle something in when I was patted down. Returning to the Formica table, I looked at the clock. It was early for me to leave to be at the prison by five, but I wanted to escape the oppressive strain of trying to jolly everyone else.

'Don't worry,' I said, as I left them. 'There's plenty of time yet. It will all work out, you watch. Keep your fingers crossed.'

'Keep your fingers crossed? It may be time to bend your knees.' Reverend Murphy Davis smiled, knowing full well she had never seen me at her church.

I smiled back and hurried off, the smile and the pretence falling away. I passed into the bright daylight.

What would I do, sitting in a room alone, waiting for someone to be killed? I carried a stack of motions that I had to file later in the week in someone's else's case. At the gate, the 'execution alert' was already in evidence. The prison was on 'code red'. They let me through without a question. I took everything out of my pockets before going inside, but for some chewing gum. My mouth gets very dry when I get nervous.

'You'll have to take that out,' the guard told me at the sign-in desk. It was a quarter of a mile back to the car. It would be easier to just get rid of it.

'Can I throw it away in your trash?' I asked, already knowing the mindless response.

'No, sir. It has to go out.' Rules are rules. 'You could leave it in the lockers inside,' she added helpfully.

'But the lockers take a quarter, and I was not meant to bring any money in,' I pointed out. To no avail.

I was early, and could not pretend there was no time. Before trekking the length of the tunnel again, I decided to go and renegotiate with Warden Zant about getting to see Larry. At the same time, perhaps I would receive a special chewing-gum dispensation. I should have known better. His idea of charity was to pull out a quarter to cut short the debate. I was powerless. I could not even pluck up the courage to indulge in petty civil disobedience: I could have jettisoned the offending spearmint in Zant's bin. Instead, I locked my gum away as I had been instructed. Eventually, I found myself in the familiar visitation area, designated for the 'inmate's witnesses'. I was the only one on the groom's side, and it was a shotgun wedding. The bride's side, with entertainment provided by the event sponsor, the warden, was for the media and other official guests, somewhere off in a more comfortable section. I had only the water fountain for company. I looked at it for want of anything else to do, wondering randomly whether the pipes were lead-soldered.

I called out on the payphone. First, I tried the number at the booth – it was busy. I was annoyed at myself for not telling them to keep it clear. I tried the main number of the diner. It was also busy. Now, I was a little scared. Finally, I tried the mobile phone – a rare commodity back then – and was relieved to hear Steve Bayliss on the other end. It had occurred to me that I had not laid out the plan for the very last moment in our defence strategy, a moment that was now approaching.

'Steve, when you talk to Larry, remember something,' I said. 'If he is strapped in the chair, he will not be able to talk because of the chin strap. He will only be able to move his hand a little. I am going to tell him when I talk to him that he should just make a thumbs up if he wants to live, and I will be there to try to get it stopped. Tell him the same thing, will you?'

Mike had called from Atlanta; he was heading to Judge Camp to get a federal court order mandating that they let me meet with Larry. Steve was suddenly indistinct. 'I think the battery's going,' were his final words. I felt as if another bank of fog was settling in, cutting me off from the shore. Unwillingly, I replaced the receiver. I looked at the motions I was working on, lying on the chair nearby. Had I really thought I would be able to concentrate on editing them at a time like this?

I went to talk with Zant again about getting to see Larry.

'I understand you've arranged some kind of hand signal with the inmate,' he accused me, before I had a chance to say anything.

I was tired, upset and slow off the mark. It did not occur to me at once that the only way he could have known was if someone in the prison had been listening in on my confidential call to Steve on the outside. So I admitted that it was true, always a mistake with people who view as criminal anything beyond breathing in 'their' prison.

'So? What am I meant to do if you won't let me speak to him? You think I'm meant to guess that he wants to live by some type of telepathy? Of course I've arranged a hand signal with him.'

'What is it?' he demanded.

'What is it?' I repeated, trying to figure out what business of his that might be.

'Yes, you're only a witness now. If you don't obey the regulations, you're out of my institution.'

'Look, I don't have to tell you. And I'm not just a witness – I'm the guy's lawyer.'

'He doesn't have a lawyer.' Zant was repeating his mantra. 'He doesn't want a lawyer, so you're not his lawyer.'

I was running into the bureaucratic brick wall that would result in my either knuckling under to some non-existent rule or being banned from the prison. The telephone rang and Zant had to answer it, momentarily distracted from trying to kick me out. It was Atlanta on the phone. I gradually understood that Judge Camp had been shocked that the prison was holding Larry incommunicado from us. The executives in the Department of Corrections had issued the edict – Larry was to be allowed constant telephone access to me in the prison. It was not contact visitation, so I could not look him in the eye, but it left Zant adrift in the bully's windless ocean – slapped down by his boss, the question of the hand signals forgotten. I was led to the internal telephone in the hallway, next to the outside line I had been using to talk to my colleagues.

Now I was faced with the awful question of what I was meant to say. I waved guards away who had no business listening to my conversation with my client, and picked up the receiver.

Larry launched into an agony of self-denigration, trying to take the blame for every evil that had happened to his family for forty years. According to him, he even managed to be the cause of my divorce from Cristiana, and my back would not be giving me problems if he was just dead and gone. I looked at my watch and saw that he had only thirty-five minutes left. I don't really remember how time passed, I have little more than an impression of a telephone line with a whole lot of emotion. I do know that I kept telling Larry that the brave thing to do was to live. But I also know what he was thinking: if he changed his mind, he would be faced with another perceived 'failure' in his life – having to walk back to death row, knowing that they believed he was not man enough to die. Meanwhile, I was not thinking clearly, and I was not coming up with many ideas.

On the outside line, I was still able to hear reports from Steve Bayliss, who had got his mobile plugged back in. He described the crumbling family. Larry had often hinted that a member of his family had somehow been involved in his crime, and that Larry had taken the rap. Now, while I had Larry crying on the phone in one ear, there were more tears in the other. Far away from the scene of the crime and the scene of the execution, one of the close relatives had promised to kill himself tonight if Larry was executed.

I hesitated for several seconds. These were extended seconds, with so few left in Larry's life. I felt wholly inadequate. What should I tell Larry and what should I hold back from him? My indecision was magnified by the week's exhaustion. If I told Larry that someone he loved would die if the execution went ahead, what might that do to Larry's last moments on earth?

True, it might tip him towards taking up his appeals, but would it not be the ultimate in emotional blackmail? If I stayed silent, I might end up being responsible for the death of two people tonight.

I was in a poker game where I had not even been dealt a complete hand, but it seemed like I had one ace.

Larry had just thirty-two minutes to live.

So I told him.

I cannot recall how I said it. I have no recollection except tears and confusion. Then I hardly understood his words when they came.

'Call it off!' he said, choking.

'What, Larry?'

'Call it off. Stop it then.'

At that moment, the phone was taken from him.

'What the hell are you doing?' I exploded, not knowing who had taken it.

'Gonna check that's what he wants,' said Marable's voice down the line, with a bitter hostility. I was split between the tentative excitement of thinking the battle was won, and a horror that Larry was exposed only to a man who so obviously wanted him to die, probably even now calling him a coward.

'Look, you've got to let me see Mr Lonchar, and right now,' I said with more conviction than I felt.

'You can't,' Marable said.

I tried to think of a reason to wrestle Larry from his grip. 'I've got to have him sign the papers to file in court.'

It was a valid reason. The petition had to be filed over his sworn signature. Yet I was surprised when Marable caved and agreed. I quickly turned to Steve on the other line, before they could change their minds. At the diner they had been looking at their watches for a long time now.

'We're OK,' I said. There was no scream of jubilation; just the sinking, deflating tension, gradually edged out by relief.

It was only moments before they brought Larry through to the visitation room. I had scribbled out a verification that he wanted a habeas petition filed in court. The sight of him was a physical slap, burning a photographic negative image into my mind that can still come palpitating back when I close my eyes. He was shaved for electrocution, the mark of Cain that showed he had been just half an hour from death. Later, I worried what my face betrayed when Larry first saw me looking at him, but he was way beyond caring. He had the crazed light in his eyes that I later saw in my nightmares. He was incoherent, one moment violently angry to be alive, the next vibratingly fearful that he had been so close to death. He signed the document I handed him without looking at it.

He handed me another piece of paper. 'Show this to the people outside,' he said. 'They gave it to me back there.'

I did not read it immediately.

I stayed with Larry for five minutes. It seemed much longer. I did not have any emotional reserve left, and I felt sure whatever I might say would be the wrong thing, or that he would take the precious authorisation back. I was actually glad when the warden told me I would have to leave. I wondered what horrors the coming night held for Larry. I promised to be back in the morning to talk to him.

I walked from the metal detector down to the tunnel that led towards the exit, surreptitiously unfolding the paper he had given me. It was a quote. I recognised where it was from.

When the executioner throws the switch that sends the electric current through the body, the prisoner cringes from torture, his flesh swells and his skin stretches to the point of breaking. He defecates, he urinates, his tongue swells and his eyes pop out. In some cases I have been told the eyeballs rest on the cheeks of the condemned. His flesh is burned and smells of cooked meat. When the autopsy is performed the liver is so hot it cannot be touched by human hand.

Justice Brennan, the most liberal of the justices on the United States Supreme Court, had penned this description a few years before, describing how the electric chair was a twentieth-century version of burning witches at the stake.

What kind of deranged person had given this to Larry? I looked around, my instinct to share my rage. A premonition that Marable would confiscate it made me push it back into my pocket. When I got to the door, I had to wait for the prison van to come and get me. I had been required to leave my car way up at the main gate of the prison. I needed to escape. I needed to be somewhere else.

But where was the sump for my repressed emotions?

By morning, Larry was miserable again. The prison placed him on suicide watch. He was furious at himself. He had come so close to escaping, yet he had lost his nerve with only half an hour to go. His enemy had become his ally, the sadistic guard who delivered that disgusting description of torture. Larry did not blame anyone but himself. His weakness was all his own.

I was trying to work out a new way to deliver hope. I had talked to the others and we had decided we could pass the hat around to pay for his father to spend more time with him – honest time. Larry looked dubious. I thought how I would feel in the same position, with my own father. Larry had strained to carry off as much of the family guilt as he could bear. Milan had been dishonest in accepting Larry's penance. His eyes shifted away, betrayed once again. I understood. After all, my father was constantly trying to get me to accept that he was in the right. Sometimes, I went along with the game to divert Dad from a more damaging tangent.

'If you're going to pay for my dad to come down to visit me,

I'd rather not,' he said. 'Instead of spending you all's money on this, give it to me. I have a friend in Vegas who will make bets for me. If you can set that up I might agree to continue this life for a year.' He said he needed $1,000. He was very precise, and had obviously been computing the numbers as we talked. I said I'd talk to the others. I wasn't sure they would go along with gambling. I wondered whether I should just pay the full sum myself, though it was more than I could afford.

In the end, I could not raise the bet. I offered a hundred myself. Larry was disappointed, and he never wanted me to spend my money. I told him that my plan involved his repaying me. I would put $100 on the Atlanta Braves baseball team to go the whole way to a World Series victory, on the promise that he could pay me when he won. I was playing Wayne Smith's role in Larry's life, but at least I was buying safety until September.

Larry went along with it. He wanted to repay me – if not in money, then in kindness.

The Braves held us together for a while, but blew it in the play-offs. Now Larry had lived hundreds of extra days, mostly in despair.

I woke up sweating. The clock read 2.06 a.m. and the night-mare was still vivid: two friends had come with me to witness Larry Lonchar's execution. It had been set for 9 p.m., but they had taken us to the chamber in vans shortly after eight. I had to travel by myself. When I got to the witness room, my friends were gone, and a group of strangers were milling around in convivial chaos. Larry was already behind the glass, pacing like an animal trapped at the zoo. He looked terrified, as he had before. He had been balding for years, and always kept what hair remained at a buzz cut. Now, somehow, he had sprouted more hair, frizzled out at angles around his ears. He started mouthing desperately to me at the glass, but I could not hear. I thought it had something to do with a debt.

I tried to sign to him. He could not understand me. I turned to a guard to be allowed in to speak in person. Miraculously, they let him out to speak with me in the witness room. His eyes were vast, covered with red veins, his speech incoherent and babbling. The people around us pushed Larry at me, as if bear-baiting. He was crazed now. Assistant Warden Marable ejected me from the witness room for causing a disturbance.

Now I was awake, it was the middle of the night, quiet, with the neon security light from the paper works on the other side of the street bright in my eyes. I could not get back to sleep.

28

Jack Kevorkian to the Rescue

My ultimate aim is to make Euthanasia a positive experience.

Jack Kevorkian

In the wake of the prison's effort to terrify him, Larry let us challenge the method of execution. When it comes to the history of the electric chair, there are various versions. In one, it is a quintessential part of Americana. Towards the end of the nineteenth century, the United States was trying to agree on a uniform grid for its electricity. Some states were also seeking an alternative to hanging – which was falling out of favour, due to various botched executions. Thomas Edison, the inventor of the light bulb, was the advocate of direct current, which was more difficult to transmit over long distances but had the advantage, he said, of being less lethal; George Westinghouse was the main proponent of alternating current. Eventually, Westinghouse won the debate, but in the 1880s the battle for the hearts and wallets of America was raging.

Although Edison was personally opposed to the death penalty, he saw the potential to increase his market share. He got his hands on a Westinghouse generator, and presented the inaugural electric chair to the state of New York as the new way of killing criminals. If Westinghouse's alternating current was seen to kill publicly, Edison hoped to impress on the citizenry the greater safety of his own electricity. The paradox spiralled down to Washington. William Kemmler, convicted for murder, was slated to be the first man executed in this new-fangled machine. Westinghouse, who was a death penalty advocate, hired the best attorneys for Kemmler to challenge the use of electrocution as a 'cruel and unusual punishment', proscribed by the Eighth Amendment. The nine justices of the Supreme Court unanimously ruled on his appeal, holding that the Constitution bars only execution methods that are 'manifestly cruel and unusual, such as burning at the stake, crucifixion, breaking on the wheel, or the like'. The punishment was certainly unusual, since Kemmler was to be its first victim, but until there was some human experimentation there could be no proof that it was sufficiently cruel.

Proponents of the novel method promised instantaneous extinction of life. In the real world, the chair malfunctioned, and it took a series of shocks to kill him. 'They would have done better using an axe,' was Westinghouse's view.

Kemmler became the charred acorn from which an oak tree of human suffering grew. The electric chair became popular across the United States as the high-tech replacement for the noose. The horror stories amplified, and another case reached the Supreme Court in 1946. The prisoner – described in the court opinion as 'Willie Francis, a colored citizen of Louisiana' – had been sentenced to death for murder. The state decided to execute Francis in the roving electric chair that was driven from parish to parish and plugged into a local generator.

Reverend Maurice Rousseve, one of the official witnesses, later described what happened. 'The executioner pulled down the switch and said, "Goodbye Willie." At that very moment, Willie Francis's lips puffed out and his body squirmed and he jumped so that the chair rocked on the floor. Then the condemned man said, "Take it off. Let me breathe."'

'I heard the one in charge yell to the man outside for more juice when he saw that Willie Francis was not dying,' reported another witness, Ignace Doucet. 'And the one on the outside yelled back he was giving him all he had . . . The boy really got a shock when they turned that machine on.' The chair failed to kill him. His lawyers argued that it would surely be cruel to allow the state another try. Francis lost his appeal, but this time the nine-member court split along the narrowest of 5–4 margins. This was, wrote the minority, 'death by instalments'. He received his second instalment the following year. Reading the appalling details of his death, I imagined Willie Francis's tortured spirit tormenting his tormentors in the deeper realms of *L'inferno*.

Fifty years later, with Larry facing Torture by Electric Chair, there had been no improvement. The same Georgia warden with whom I had been crossing swords had recently tried to kill Otis Stephens. After the first two jolts, the doctors had to wait six minutes until his body cooled sufficiently for them to check for life signs. 'Mr Stephens took about 23 breaths. At 12.26 a.m., two doctors examined him and said he was alive,' the *New York Times* reported. 'A second two-minute charge was administered at 12.28 a.m.'

Why did it take so long? Mr Stephens 'was just not a conductor of electricity', a Georgia prison official said.

While we sued to try to abolish the chair forever, Larry fluctuated. Then he dropped his appeals again. I found us – Larry and me – within four days of his execution once more. That was when I got a call from Dr Death himself, Jack Kevorkian. America is often a single-issue society, and Jack's was euthanasia. His mantra was 'dying is not a crime': we each have the right to 'self-deliverance', and he offered to pole us across the River Styx in the good punt *Patholysis*. When he started talking about harvesting organs, Jack made me feel differently about the autumn harvest festival.

From his website, I learned that Jack was an amateur artist as well as a pathologist. *Nearer My God to Thee* showed a desperate man slipping towards death, five parallel nail tracks tracing each hand down the brick walls of doom. There was an advertisement for Jack's professional services. 'If you or someone you know wants to die, call Jack Kevorkian.' I could almost hear a jolly American tone. 'He's the best.' For all his self-hype, I respected Jack's effort to provoke contentious moral debate. However, it was with some trepidation that I wondered whether Jack could give Larry a reason to live.

I picked up the telephone with my prejudices securely intact. I imagined his well-known gaunt face on the other end of the line, his thin, sharp features shrouded in grey around the eyes. He was a charming man, insisting that I call him Jack. He was not in favour of the death penalty. He referred repeatedly to the barbarism of our society; one area where we could surely all find common ground was electrocution. For someone intent on harvesting organs, electrocution was, he said, worse than mad cow disease: no organs could be used. 'If you kill people with lethal injection,' he told me clinically, 'you can still use the kidneys and liver if they are taken out immediately. You can't use the heart and lungs, though. They're poisoned.'

Rather than lethal poisons, Jack envisioned execution by surgery. Every day in America, Jack told me, eight people die for lack of an available organ. 'You see, to be both compassionate and sensible, executions should really be carried out as surgical procedures,' he continued. 'The surgeon puts the condemned man under with a rapid anaesthesia that puts him out for about ten minutes. Then we use regular gas anaesthesia to take the organs. Obviously, by the time you have lost your heart and lungs you are dead anyway, and that is the end of it.'

Jack was in his element. 'Up to ten people's lives could be saved by the donation of the organs,' he explained, with zeal tingling the telephone. 'The heart, that's one; the lungs, two and three; kidneys, four and five; the liver, that could be two more if it were split for babies; the pancreas, small intestine and bone marrow, eight, nine and ten. Ten lives saved for one that society has said it's going to take anyway.' *Lex talionis* times ten.

So very simple. There was the minor matter of the Hippocratic oath – which doctor would do it? – along with the real-life vision of a queue of desperate people on life support waiting impatiently for their chance at Larry's innards. I imagined the pressure on the elected justices of the Georgia Supreme Court asked to issue a stay minutes away from the execution of a reviled murderer, with the lives of half a dozen organ recipients hanging in the balance. I voiced a few of my concerns, though I was careful to pose them as possible media snags that might come up in our joint campaign. After all, my goal was rather limited: preventing Larry from destroying himself in the coming days. Jack could be the solution here, and I did not want to offend him.

I sold the Kevorkian idea to Larry as best I could. Jack Kevorkian and I might have had different goals – he was going to collect some organs and kill Larry, I wanted Larry to live – but the immediate problem was to keep Larry alive for the next few hours and days. He had, as ever, painted himself inexorably into a corner, but here was a way to prove that it took more courage for him to live than to die – at least until Jack was allowed to start using his scalpel. The idea of atoning for his sins by saving ten lives inevitably appealed to Larry. Larry wanted nothing more than to get out of the confines of the Georgia Diagnostic and Classification Center. It seemed rather desperate to escape in increments – first a kidney, before moving on to more vital organs. Like Humpty Dumpty, it might not be so easy to put him back together again.

The flood of calls had already begun from the West Coast. I hoped Larry was tuned in from his prison cell. He was on television, all over. The story was no longer about people gunned down in an Atlanta condo. Now, at last, the media was talking about something else: how many lives he could save. Yet if Larry was edging towards us – he was not yet there – we had an enemy within. The execution ritual tends to attract people who find it exciting, and the only people who do are on the fringes of good sense.

Her name was Sondra London. It is difficult to do her justice on the written page and her website appears to have changed of late. When I first visited, I encountered a particularly vampish picture, captioned with her life philosophy: 'It is good to know the truth, but it is better to speak of palm trees.' She still boasted that she was the 'Queen of Serial-Killer Journalism', but now preferred to highlight her 'pioneering work with the late Discordian Nonprophet Kerry Thornley', putting him on national TV for his conspiracy theories regarding the assassination of JFK.

I had first come across Sondra some years earlier in her role as the self-proclaimed 'Editor of the Damned', where she spread the writings of serial killers in prison across the page. Sondra never meant anyone ill, she was just peculiar. This may have had roots in high school, where she had been sweetheart to a future mass killer, Gerard Schaefer – reputed to have murdered as many as thirty-four women in the 1970s. They had drifted apart after the high-school prom, but her web page subsequently featured advice from Keith Jesperson, the 'Happy Face Killer' who signed letters confessing to various murders with smiley faces. His writings included a 'self-start serial-killer kit', helpfully promoted as a way 'to get rid of that unwanted family member'.

At one point her résumé listed her fiancé as Danny Rolling, the son of a Shreveport police officer. Rolling ended up on the lethal injection gurney for killing several women in their college dormitories. Five years before, when Sondra first wafted, heavily perfumed, into my life, Danny had been writing a novel. As his editor, Sondra pointed out that his *tragediennes* were invariably thin on character, entering the book for a page or two and then dying in a gory throat-slashing. Sondra suggested ways to improve his prose – perhaps he could practise writing letters in the guise of his female protagonists? Danny therefore imagined himself to be a profoundly perverse woman who wrote letters to various men on Virginia's death row, including my client Joe O'Dell, with a description of the orgasm that she would enjoy while watching them fry in the electric chair. Because he could not put his prison address on the envelopes, Danny's letters originated from Sondra's home, and she received the replies. I was proud of Joe: he merely told Danny's heroine to leave him alone. Some of the other recipients were less temperate. She wept into the telephone: could I ask Joe to call off the other baying wolves who were threatening her with all kinds of slashings themselves? My next call came from an FBI agent who explained, tiredly, how Sondra had put Danny up to this.

Nothing (at least nothing tasteful) had come of it all, and it was on the edges of my memory. I had not heard from her for a while. Now, like the turbid oil that roiled the waves after the *Torrey Canyon* disaster, she came gushing back in. She had agreed, she proudly announced, to witness Larry's final moments and write up his story. Two days before his scheduled death, unbeknown to me, Sondra had managed to get in to see him. Larry had been glad of the excuse to get into the air-conditioned visitors' room and away from his cell. She had produced examples of her purple prose: she would do justice to his death.

'When they strap me in, I will be calm,' she began, declaiming her proposed posthumous statement. 'I might be crying a little bit but it's not because of fear. It's just because I'll miss my mommy.' She demonstrated how she would read it to the awaiting media after his death. She would smile gravely into the cameras. She knew how frightening the chair was, she said, and this would cover for Larry if the press witnesses thought they saw any signs of terror. Her seduction was a brimming mug of Dutch courage held out to slake the thirst of suicide. If she got in to see him again today, I wondered whether she would secure an exclusive contract, and have Larry exclude not just me, but everyone else as well.

That morning, due to be the penultimate in Larry's life, I got up early and arrived at the prison before her, to monopolise the visiting room as best I could. While I was there, the prison might not allow other visitors in. It was to be my last, depressing meeting with Larry. He had told the prison I was to be banned after ten o'clock today to prevent me from talking him around. We had arranged other options, other lawyers who knew him, but his prohibition against my visits would kick in when I left, and I did not have the heart to ask him to change it. I had done enough to hurt Larry; it would hurt him more to deny me a final wish. I had to leave. It was another farewell.

Larry told me about his conversation with Sondra, and wondered out loud whether her lurid writing would ever get published. I sensed that disenchantment had already begun to set in with his post-mortem spokesperson. As I walked, sombre, out of the prison, I wanted only to get in my car and drive. Instead, I encountered an irate Sondra in the parking lot, sputtering angrily towards the guard tower. Reluctantly, I approached, noticing a teenager behind her, considerably under half her age.

'He's my sex slave,' said Sondra, seeing my glance. She smiled through her melting make-up. He smirked weakly through his adolescent acne. She explained she had just been banned from the prison. She had failed to make an appointment. She projected every insult she could muster at the guard in the tower. She pleaded with me to intervene. I did call the warden, but – I must confess my hypocrisy – only to express my sympathy and reassure him that Sondra had no official link to my office. His intransigence was a divine intervention.

Sondra truly meant to be an ally. I was relieved when she departed, sweating, in a swathe of black pseudo-satin.

Just before the family was due to be thrown out of the prison, four hours before the current would be turned on, it came.

Larry had signed something. He wanted Jack Kevorkian to harvest his organs. Miraculously, we had a stay until Tuesday morning, four full days hence, when the state judge would consider a permanent stay.

It was Friday. Nothing would happen over the weekend. It is difficult, in the midst of battle, to lay down arms and do nothing. That afternoon, Larry had had just four hours to live; now he had four days, an age. Ten years before, I would have found it impossible to sleep. I could not have permitted myself pause until I had dragged the client, both of us exhausted, safely out of the quicksand sucking him down to the Chair. But life had become a succession of these moments. The monstrous had become mundane. My adrenaline stocks were running low.

The shroud of guilt gradually lifting as I drove, I went to the hills of North Carolina to meet my friend David Utter for a few beers and a game of golf at his father's holiday house. The family was on vacation together, swapping stories of the country crafts they had seen that day; I surfaced, shell-shocked, from one of the trenches at the Somme. I dissociated, set it all aside, borrowed some clubs and headed to the course.

On Monday, David and I were preparing to slice our drives on the twenty-seventh hole of the day when his father came out towards the fairway with a worried expression. Judge Smith had ruled a day early, lifting the stay and setting the execution for Wednesday, at 3 p.m. I took a swing, imagining the ball were an elected official. The ball nestled deep among the distant trees.

The next day, Tuesday, we moved on to federal court. Some might say that we were four days ahead of the game – had it not been for the stay at the end of the previous week, Larry would have been cold in his grave now, albeit once his blood had been brought to boiling point in the electric chair. Judge Camp let me talk as much as I wanted, as I cast furtive glances at the courtroom clock. When I was through, he probed me with some difficult questions. Not satisfied even then, he made me take the stand as a witness. He was struggling to decide whether Larry could truly have 'waived' his right to federal review of his case. Nobody had actually told Larry that if he dropped his appeals *this* time then he would never be permitted to return. I had always been keenly aware of this, and had been very careful with what I had said.

'What advice did you give to Mr Lonchar?' Assistant Attorney General Mary Beth Westmoreland asked, when the prosecution got their chance at me.

'I told Larry that he would always get a stay,' I replied, trying to think how best to encourage Judge Camp to do the right thing. I told the whole story, as completely as I could. 'I told him that he ought to get a stay in state court, but quite honestly political considerations might come between him and justice in a court where judges are elected.'

Mary Beth tried to cut me off. I held up my hand. I was not finished.

'I told Larry that an Article III judge' – Judge Camp was guaranteed life tenure by the Federal Constitution – 'would not play politics. I told him that he would get a stay in federal court, once he got there.' Judge Camp obviously disapproved of the way that Larry had come to his court, but he had sworn an oath himself to uphold the law, and the law did not allow him to dismiss Larry's case out of hand. He finally entered a temporary stay. He would rule on our request for a longer injunction that evening, he said.

'Judge, may we brief the issues?' I asked tentatively. We were ahead, and I did not want to wreck it.

'How long do you need?' he asked politely.

'That depends on how good a brief you want,' I replied. 'I'll settle for whatever time you give us.'

'Very well,' he said, thinking for a moment. 'Get me what you can by three thirty.' I scrambled to a car. Mike Mears paused for a moment with the press at the front door of the courthouse to tell them how Judge Camp had made a judicious decision. The rules of his robe left him unable to defend himself, so it became our duty to stand in for him.

The memorandum was in with a couple of minutes to spare, and the phoney war began once more. We waited, and nothing

307

happened. It was nine o'clock that night and I was alone in the office. I was too tired to get much useful done, but with the tension still building I was far from sleep. The others had taken my advice and left, but I was still preparing for the worst, working on an appeal and stay motion to the court of appeals.

Judge Camp's clerk called.

'The order is coming through on the fax now,' she said.

'Can you tell me what it says?' There was a pause while she thought about the propriety of this. I could not see what was wrong with telling me the words that were already snaking through the telephone line towards our fax. 'I only want to know the last word.'

'OK. *Denied*,' she said, reading. I was so used to 'DENIED' that I was momentarily disappointed. Then I realised that it was the state's motion, so the state was on the losing end of the word for once. 'Motion to dismiss denied.'

'Thanks,' I said. 'You just made my evening.' I called around to tell everyone. Nobody was answering. They were either dead to the world or out and trying to ignore the chaos around them.

I got eight hours of sleep that night.

'We need not pause to consider whether this should properly be deemed an abuse of the writ, or merely abusive conduct,' the Eleventh Circuit Court of Appeals wrote the next afternoon. They were just mad at Larry for what they viewed as toying with them: he should lose and be executed. The mandate (which would give the state of Georgia authority to plug the Chair in) would issue at five o'clock and Larry could be executed at seven. Just like that. There was no discussion in their short opinion of anything that had happened before Judge Camp the day before. The opinion had obviously been in the works before Judge Camp had even held a hearing.

I looked at the fax. By the time it arrived it was 3.02 p.m. Larry had just three hours and fifty-eight minutes to live.

Visitation had ended punctiliously at three, so Larry's mother would have left, under the genial illusion that Larry was safe; she had missed saying goodbye to him by two minutes.

We were stunned. Mike Mears sat staring watery-eyed at the ceiling. Steve Bayliss watched the back of his hand. Laura Patton turned to the floor. Nobody moved. We had won in front of a conservative district court judge only to have it snatched from us by the appeals court, which was generally more liberal.

Just in case the state bothered to appeal to the Supreme Court, I had been writing an opposition. As the shock wore off, I started a skim-edit to change it to an application for the Supreme Court to hear the case.

The second hand on my watch was ticking loudly. Larry's life was ebbing by the second, each an immense increment, yet the petition was due in minutes that were hopelessly short. I knew that the Supreme Court was likely itching to kill Larry. From their perspective, he had messed with them too many times – and while not very judicial, their attitude is human enough: there were more than *3,000* men and women sentenced to die in the United States, and each one would apply to the Supreme Court for relief six to ten times. With half of the court over seventy years old, the very idea of 20,000 applications must be draining.

Cynicism leaves room to doubt how much attention the justices are able to pay to these last-minute papers, so I had taken to addressing them like a kindergarten class, highlighting the most important points:

- Larry Lonchar is about to become the first person since 1972 to be denied even one round of appeals.
- Neither the prosecution nor the court of appeals could find *one* case in support of their position.
- The same people who now say that Larry is calculating and manipulative have admitted for five years that he is mentally ill.

I skimmed through it and recognised how much better it could have been. This was the last appeal in Larry's life. This was the Supreme Court of the United States, nine of the most powerful people in the country. I was momentarily angry that I was forced to write a fifth-rate plea in a matter of minutes, but there was no time to change it. As it printed, I prayed that there would not be a jam. At least these days I could fax it, rather than having to fly up to Washington to file it. The Supreme Court clerk, Frank Larson, had told me the petition had to be in by five. As it was, the printer did not jam, the fax ran smoothly, and it arrived in Washington with one hundred and twenty seconds to spare. Larry was a few hours from death for the third time in a week.

There were one hundred and twenty minutes left of his life. If I jumped in my car right now, I could be at the prison with an hour to spare. They would let me in, right back to the visitation area, to sit alone and wait to watch Larry die. It already seemed so long ago, but I had watched another man, Nicky Ingram, die in the same electric chair eighty-three days before. I ought to go again.

I had looked up post-traumatic stress disorder in the *DSM* : nightmares, intrusive memories, irrational reactions to people with shaven heads . . . I could not go down to the prison to witness Larry's execution. When I had watched men die before, I had known how I would react, within parameters. I had known that I would be able to hold myself together. I did not know now.

I admitted to the others that I could not go. Nobody else was eager to take my place.

Larry would die alone.

I was paralysed, sure that I could not go to the prison, but equally certain that I would always regret letting Larry down. I could not face speaking to Warden Zant to ask for the collect call, with them now so close to achieving Larry's death. I asked Steve Bayliss to do it. A few minutes later, the phone rang.

'This is AT&T with a collect call to anybody from . . .' intoned the automated message, leaving a pause for the prisoner to state his name. 'Larry Lonchar.' The recorded voice was tired, dull with resignation.

'To accept . . .' continued the voice. We had been through this rigmarole many times. I pressed '1' before the computer told me to.

'Hey, Larry,' I said.

'This the lawyer?' asked a voice. A guard was checking that this was a proper attorney call. 'Hold on while I get Mr Lonchar.' I was pleased to hear the respect for Larry.

'Hello?' Larry said, not sure who it was. I knew he would be expecting news. I had none.

'Hey, Larry, it's me, Clive.'

'What's going on, then, Clive?' he asked, listless.

'We just filed in the Supreme Court,' I said. 'I wanted you to know.'

'Yeah,' he said. I had been to see him early that morning. He had been optimistic, glad that Judge Camp saw sufficient merit in him as a human being for a stay. All the expression had now drained from his voice. 'No chance there, is there?'

'Yes, Larry, we've got a chance. A good chance. You know, it was a hell of a stay motion, if I say so myself. The law's all on our side.' I said it as if I meant it.

'Nah. Clive, you know them in Washington, they're the worst of all of them. You know the Eleventh Circuit's always been the best hope. The Supreme Court ain't gonna do anything.' It was hard to argue with him. 'M-a-a-a-n,' Larry went on, depression reeking down the phone line. 'It's just the way my life's always been. I wanted to die for seven years – seven fucking years!' For a moment, anger replacing desolation. 'And they wouldn't do it for me. First time now, you guys have given me a reason to want to live, and here they are gonna kill me. Man, I can't believe that. You had me so optimistic this morning,' he said without recrimination. 'I never even started my letters goodbye. Now I don't have time to get them all done. You know what a trouble I have putting words together. No way I can get them all done. No way.'

A pause.

'But it was good, though,' he went on. 'Mom, when she left, she was all happy, 'cause we all thought it was gonna work out OK. It's all for the best, really. But I'd better write what I can.' His voice trailed off towards one of his typical troughs. Selfishly, I was glad he had something he wanted to do. It was impossible to think of anything to say, to have any meaningful conversation, with someone headed towards the electric chair. I promised to make sure, if he did not get his letters done in time to die, that everyone got his goodbyes. It was one of the strange promises that an execution brings on us. We hung up, with me saying I'd call as soon as there was news to tell.

I had not even had the courage to tell him that I would not be there for him. But Larry knew. He knew all of these things. He knew that I was just another person who had let him down in the end.

When I put down the receiver, we were at ninety-two minutes. There was nothing to do but pace about, pull a beer out of the fridge, and pretend that the world was not a wasteland. Alcohol does not mix with complex decisions, but the choices were all in the past. Mike had run out. He returned with more beer and a small book of poetry that he had promised me two days before – a collection of poems by W. H. Auden. I turned to the old favourite, 'Funeral Blues' ('Stop all the clocks . . . '). Larry may not ever have understood it, but he had been every point on the compass to his mother. Her favourite son about to die a terrible death.

And I thought, tears welling, of what Larry meant to me. I had never had a friend who had trusted me to go where Larry had taken me. Yet I could not avoid the accusing finger of my conscience. I was not down at the prison for him now. I was sitting on the floor in the office, staring at the desk in front of me, half aware of the muted muttering around me.

Just before half past six, a call came through from Washington.

'You got anything else you're going to file?' asked Frank Larson, the clerk.

'No,' I said. 'That's all.'

I knew what that meant. That was shorthand. There would be an execution. If something else was needed, that meant that we had not sent enough. Another clerk had asked the same question in Nicky Ingram's case less than three months before. After that coded call, it had been just half an hour before I was in the clinging atmosphere of the witness room, watching as the guards strapped Nicky into the electric chair.

I didn't tell anyone what Frank had said. No point in dragging everyone down before I had to.

'No news from the Supremes,' I said, when they asked me. 'Still just waiting.'

In the room next door, I could hear the others patching Larry through on the phone to Arnold, a friend of his in New York. He had quit writing his farewells. It must have been desperately lonely – shaven and waiting. He was saving paper. Maybe the Supreme Court would hold off until close to seven o'clock, before we heard the Damoclean *Denied*.

Outside the half-closed door, the office was crowded with the other people – lawyers, investigators, summer students, everyone supporting each other. I wanted to be alone, away from the false optimism, alone with my knowledge that the code had been spoken. I would have to bear Larry the final verdict. It would be a lie for me to cheer him up now, when I already knew the outcome. There is a thin line between good intentions and outright hypocrisy. I wondered morosely how many times I had crossed that line with Larry in the past seven years.

With twelve minutes of life left, draining through the hour-glass, I got nervous and reached for the telephone.

'You heard anything?' I had called Mary Beth Westmoreland, the state's lawyer. I almost expected her to say that the Supreme Court had turned us down. The state always hears first, and earlier that day she had let me know of the Eleventh Circuit's ruling before they bothered to tell us.

'No, nothing,' she said. I was relieved. I needed that infinitesimal illusion myself. For a few more minutes.

'Well, let me know if anything changes, will you, so I can try to get some kind of emergency stay?'

'Yes, I'll give you a call if anything comes up.'

I hung up. Silence for a minute, two minutes.

Frank Larson came on the line again.

'Frank, what's going on? It's only seven minutes to go.'

'What's the best line for you?' he asked.

'The 898-2060 number. 404 area code.'

'Make sure nobody gets on it, OK?'

'Of course,' I said. 'The state says they will wait to hear from you—'

'I heard—'

'But let me know the moment you have anything.'

'I will.' And he hung up. Everyone looked at me, questioning. I shook my head. Nothing.

Silence.

Someone else was still doing telephone duty with Larry in the office next door. I closed my door to be alone with the phone, counting down the seconds to it ringing. I remembered the same moment years before, on 21 May 1987, when I had to deliver the final message to Edward Johnson. Wanting it to be over, but wanting above all else for the telephone never to ring.

I should be down there. Larry needed to have one friend at his side.

6.57. Three minutes to go. I could wait no longer. I called

Washington, the number now coming automatically to my fingers. Frank answered.

'What is it, Frank?' I asked.

'Can you wait a minute?' he replied.

I was about to say that I couldn't when the line went silent, and I realised that I was on hold. The bookshelf on the other side of the office began to spiral. The phone felt ethereal, the untouchable messenger of death.

6.58.50. Seventy seconds to go. Silence.

6.59. Sixty seconds. They might make Larry hang up any moment.

The phone came alive. I could feel Frank on the other end. I did not have time to ask.

'Stay granted. Cert granted. Eight to one, Rehnquist dissenting.' That was all he said.

Later, I realised I might have been rude. I was numb. I'm not sure if I even thanked him before I hung up. I likely did. Many years of English indoctrination probably made it automatic. But it bothered me later not to be sure.

I stumbled to my feet, a couple of beers on a three-day-empty stomach catching me at the ankles. 'Stay granted, cert granted,' I told everyone as I went to the other phone. Silence. They understood, of course – the court had not only stayed the execution, but granted certiorari: the full Supreme Court had agreed to hear Larry's case up in Washington, some day well into the future. The chances of having a case heard are minuscule. Larry's was that one in two hundred. His number had come up at last.

'Stay granted, cert granted.' It was a mantra by the time I said the words into Larry's phone, where he sat nervously on the other end. The tears of emotion finally breaking through the wall of silence.

'What's that mean?' Larry said, after a moment of silence.

'It means we've won, Larry, it means we've won.' That was

all I could say. As I said it, something made me look at my watch. The second hand had just ticked past seven. I was on the verge of sobbing without control. I had to end the conversation quickly. 'I'll come down and tell you what it means in the morning.'

In the morning. Larry would have another morning. I could barely get out a see-you-later before I passed the phone to someone else who would be able to talk to Larry more coherently.

29

Forgiveness

> I am the master of my fate:
> I am the captain of my soul.
>
>   William Ernest Henley, 'Invictus'

I visited Dad in his little flat in Ely on one of my trips back to the UK. He had once been obsessed with his height – he was, he used to say, six feet tall, when he was actually five-eleven and a half, as if a tiny distinction in an arbitrary measurement system was the key to his manhood. Now, he was definitively diminutive, no more than five-four. His back had simply collapsed, his spinal column crushing down on itself. He was in pain most days. He seemed so very small.

Still fixated on tourism as the future for all society's ills, Dad had recently had one of his imaginative ideas that might have been a success with the right 'implementation'. It was something he called Photofit – both a good scheme and a good name to go with it. He had pored over a collection of 250,000 old illustrations of various towns. He would use centuries-old pictures of a place such as Cambridge or Ely, sold with a cheap instant camera. A visitor would take a tour, armed with a small guidebook with stories that detailed the historical significance of each landmark. The challenge would be to take a contemporary photograph at precisely the same angle as the original, and return a complete collection at the end of the day, with a prize for the best. It was the kind of thing that would work even better today, with an app on a smartphone that could instantaneously grade each picture for angles and accuracy.

'Fortunately, you see, I met a young guy on the bus to Bury on Tuesday who I would be proud to count among my sons and who would justify the nickname "Chip",' he told me. He had taken to calling me Chip, as I was a chip off the old block. I disliked it immensely, though I did not tell him as it would only have encouraged him in its use. 'I mean, he's the ideal guy to run Photofit and is ardent to do so.' He opined that the project would be making £200,000 a year in two years. Sadly, this Chip was yet another of the endless casualties, and Photofit never made it off the runway. If I had spent a tenth of the time I devoted to Larry helping Dad to achieve something through Photofit, it might have happened. It might never have made millions, but it would have given him satisfaction.

Dad was slowing down, but still writing letters – as 'an applied theologian' – to everyone in the Church of England, about the need to stave off Britain's moral decline, much of which was apparently traceable directly to St Paul. Dad was high again, though he was running out of energy to do as much harm. A current indicator was the range of prelates who were receiving his letters: bishops and archbishops. 'I received and read your contribution with appreciation,' the Archbishop of Canterbury wrote. 'I do think you are pretty rotten about St Paul. After all, some of the most beautiful language in the Bible about faith, hope and love, certainly does not fit into your caricature! But I am afraid we had better agree to differ on this without engaging in more lengthy correspondence.'

The Bishop of Lambeth quickly got Dad's measure and replied only once; when he bowed out, it was the Bishop of Chichester's turn, followed by the bishops of Norwich, Durham, Edinburgh, Leicester, Brixworth, Lynn and Ely. I had no idea where Brixworth was or how it came to have a bishop. The Reverend Jeremy Martineau, archdeacon to the Bishop of Leicester, was the kindest of them all. He sent Dad £200 for 'travelling expenses' – simple charity.

Dad was elated. 'Two hundred in the post!' he told Mum. 'The start of an avalanche. The "victory" yesterday may not seem a major triumph but in fact it represents far more than the immediate outcome of seeing me eat and work over Easter – though that in itself is of no small significance viewed from where I sit!'

Sadly, within two months, he wrote – starting the letter at 5 a.m. on a Sunday – that Martineau had failed Dad's impossible test. 'Whose morality is going to govern the joint project and the Church from now on?' he demanded of the Bishop of Leicester. 'Yours and the archdeacon's with its double standards and lack of driving enthusiasm, or mine with the integrity and efficiency of the true professional?' It is difficult to see what he expected to achieve by this.

'I do not feel it would be helpful for me to meet you,' the bishop inevitably replied.

Dad was also sending regular missives to the *Daily Telegraph*, all of which fortunately remained unpublished. One focused on his expectations of the afterlife. 'May I, through your columns and writing as an applied scientific theologian, add one further thought to the current debate on the meaning of hell?' he wrote. 'I believe that after death – or possibly after an initial cup of tea to help with the shock of being "on the other side"! – we are placed before a screen and given the opportunity to watch a replay of our lives showing all the things which would have happened had we done all the things which we ought to have done but did not do and had we not done all the things we did but ought not to have done. Can you imagine a worse form of hell than that for anyone with a conscience?'

I thought Dad's deepening obsession with religion and the afterlife grew out of his fear of meaninglessness. Yet, far away in the bayous surrounding New Orleans, I was finally learning a rather elementary lesson: I should look for the best in everyone, rather than disparaging them. If I wanted to identify and draw on the best of the jurors before me, I had to speak the language they understood. In the Deep South that meant Christianity.

When I had first tried a case, far too soon after I left a British public school, I did what came naturally to me – when I wanted the jurors to show mercy, I quoted *The Merchant of Venice*: 'The quality of mercy is not strain'd, it droppeth as the gentle rain from heaven.' The north Georgia jurors looked at me as if I had dropped from an alien planet. An elderly local lawyer, Bobby Lee Cook, had come up after my closing argument and gently educated me.

'These here jurors wouldn't know who William Shakespeare was!' he exclaimed. 'I've used that selfsame passage myself, but when I did I began by saying, "I think it was in the Book of Job I read." Then I'd quote it. That way it was somethin' they understood.'

He did laugh at himself, and admit that the prosecutor had called him up after one trial, three sheets to the wind, and said, 'Bobby Lee! I've read that the-yar Book of Job *three times* an' it ain't in there!'

It was a chastening lesson. I was speaking the wrong language. Once I understood this, capital cases became much easier. I do not retreat from my personal beliefs: I confess that I think the notion that some god sent his son down to this planet is about as silly an idea as one could conjure up. Yet there is a distinction between a bizarre belief and one that is somehow dangerous. It was my mistake to allow my prejudices to prevent me from seeking out the best in others. Christians (and others who believe in such things) have some remarkably generous beliefs. For them, a capital case really comes down to one verse of the Bible – Matthew 5:7. 'Blessed are the Merciful, for they shall obtain mercy.' If the jurors want to get to heaven they must show mercy; if they do as the prosecutor demands, they are asking for eternal damnation.

Or, I learned to invite the jurors to think 'W W J D?' in their deliberations. There would be the twelve of them in the jury room sharing their views, I said, but what if there was a thirteenth juror – Jesus Christ? What would Jesus do? Could they truly imagine that he would demand that they should 'fry the motherfucker'?

If we asked the man on the Clapham Omnibus to name the worst crime a human can commit, he would likely say some form of murder. A Pentecostal juror would say that even murder could be forgiven, but failing to accept Jesus as your Lord and Saviour could not. Yet a Pentecostal juror would translate the *DSM* into a different language: alcoholism was Satan grabbing the ankles of the clients, dragging them down. If my client was himself Christian, the jurors were not showing pity or sympathy; they were *empathising*, because they recognised the client's human traits.

Christianity – and other religions – may be the opiate of the masses, but opiates have many positive uses. Indeed, I would legalise all drugs.

30

Larry Lonchar: The Finale

Once more unto the breach, dear friends, once more;
Or close the wall up with our English dead!
William Shakespeare, *Henry V* (Act III, Scene 1)

13 November 1996. A Wednesday, not a Friday, but nevertheless unlucky. He was electrocuted just after midnight.

I had spent eight years struggling with Larry's self-destruction, and finally he had won his death. I had prolonged his misery through eight torrid summers, where the whir of fans on death row had pushed the suffocating heat from one cell to another and back again. By now, everyone seemed to hate him: the public thought him manipulative, the men on the row thought he was a coward, and even his family seemed almost glad that the ordeal was over.

Larry's execution was perhaps the most reaffirming experience of my life to date. I had been able to witness for him.

The guards brought Larry into the death chamber and began to strap him in. Larry looked out to the front. Although he was held down by six large, close-shaved and heavyset officers, he managed to wave to me with the fingers of his left hand. He was calm. I had feared his fear more than anything else. Larry had always been so afraid of the electric chair, and yet this evening he showed none of it.

The new warden, Tony Turpin, asked Larry if he had any last words. It was Turpin's first execution.

Larry hesitated. 'Yes,' he said, with only a slight tremor in his voice. He looked up to the ceiling, as he often did. 'Lord, forgive them, for they know not what they do.'

The other thirty-three witnesses looked down at their feet in unison. They knew the echo. Though they might later insist that Larry was no Jesus Christ, they would never escape the accusing finger: they were just the rabble in front of the Cross, baying for blood.

Larry had written a longer final statement, but he did not want to try to declaim it. He left that for me to read out when the execution was over.

To God: thank you for loving me so much that you sent your Son to die for me.

To my family and the victims: I have caused so much pain and tears. I am so deeply sorry.

To the people of the state of Georgia: thank you for killing me. You thought you was punishing me. Instead you rewarded me by sending me to a better place, heaven. Jesus Christ died for my sins too. Since I recently accepted the fact that Jesus Christ is my Saviour, I now know God gave me a reason the times my execution was scheduled to stop it, because I wasn't ready to spend eternity with Him. He knows now, like I do, I am ready and will be with Him forever so, again, thank you people of the state of Georgia.

A simple question to the people who think they are Christians but believe the Bible supports Capital Punishment: would Jesus Christ push the buttons tonight that kill me?

Back in the execution chamber, the show had to go on.

'Would you like a final prayer?' Warden Turpin intoned to Larry, following the script. When Larry said yes, that was his last audible word on this earth. I was glad that they had brought in the black prison minister. I did not know his name, but Larry had said he was the decent one.

'Let us pray for our friend Larry Lonchar. Let us pray that our friend and brother in Christ passes from this world into a better one . . .' I did notice the anomaly as it floated past me – Larry was our friend, yet we were about to kill him right there in front of us. He was my friend. Then my mind slipped away, and I don't know what else the minister said. I hoped the prayer would go on forever, and yet I hoped it would soon be finished.

There were a number of witnesses. Apparently they wanted to be present. Bob Wilson, once a foe of the death penalty, had been the district attorney in charge of Larry's prosecution before he ran for Congress. Larry's scalp was a trophy in his political campaigns. He had spent the previous few minutes studiously avoiding me. Even the journalists averted their eyes.

Twelve minutes later, Larry was dead. Seven hundred and twenty seconds – try saying 'Mississippi' that many times and you will understand how long it can be. I stopped watching when they pulled the leather mask over his face. My job was done. If Larry could not see me, then there was no point in my watching his final agony.

And it was agony. The chair 'malfunctioned' as it had with Otis Stephens. Maybe Larry was not a good conductor. Maybe, after all Larry had put them through, some prison sadist had used the wrong water in the sponge so it would not pass a proper current.

I closed my eyes in my hands, and waited for the angry buzz of electricity to be over.

Larry had lived another seventeen months after the United States Supreme Court took his case. He made a little history – *Lonchar* v. *Thomas*, a unanimous victory with the nine justices in Washington. For the death row inmate, this was a rare occurrence these days. The court had reversed the Eleventh Circuit's ruling, recognising Larry's right to proceed with his case. He would have won his appeal outright – and been given a new trial – if only he had allowed it.

But Larry's bipolar roller coaster had taken in several crests and troughs in that year and a half. He had periodically sent me a message that he wanted to drop his appeals and die. Each time he would try to place increasingly impossible conditions on my continuing to represent him. Eventually, he wrote me a kind letter, including a copy of his handwritten motion to the judge asking that his appeals be dropped. The Atlanta Olympics were just over, and Georgia had shed its shame over executions.

Two weeks later we were in court before Judge Camp at a hearing to determine the voluntariness of his choice. I had a go at the psychiatrist, Dave Davis, who was still getting paid for helping to push Larry into oblivion. But when Larry testified, I did not cross-examine him. He wanted to die. He would not say why. He did not want any more appeals. He understood that this would be his last chance. We knew the routine. We had been there before several times. In his testimony, he had not been forthright about half a dozen things, but I was not going to accuse Larry of lying in public. Larry would never embarrass me in front of my enemies, and there was honour between us. He'd painted himself into a corner. It was going to be impossible to get him out.

Larry had become a Christian. We talked about it.

'What they say's gotta be true,' he said, looking at me stead-fastly. He genuinely believed, although his rationale was not directly out of the catechism. 'I know snitches. Twelve of them, the Apostles, and eleven got executed for him.'

'Eleven?' I did not mean to interrupt Larry's explanation, but I could not help asking, wondering if he meant Judas Iscariot.

'John,' Larry explained. 'He died of old age. Eighty-something. He was the only one didn't get executed.' He looked up at me again. This was a very different experience. Larry would normally either stare at the floor or let his eyes wander aimlessly across the ceiling as you talked.

'All the other eleven let themselves be killed,' he went on. 'All they had to do to save themselves was renounce him. Even if they believed, most people would've said that to save their lives. I know snitches. Most people'd do that even if they thought it was true. You've gotta believe it if eleven of them went down. Eleven out of twelve.'

I sat there, watching him as he repeated himself. With every repetition he was winning the argument with himself: faith founded on fact. My natural instinct was to argue with him. Seeing him so calm for the first time in eight years, I held my tongue. I had nothing against opiates; Larry had found one that would neutralise the suffering of the Diagnostic Center. I had no alternative prescription. I had made enough decisions in Larry's life. Larry had teetered on the ledge eight years ago, and I had pulled him back in. He had tried to jump several times since, and I had grabbed him. This time I knew I could not hold on to him. Larry was about to find out first-hand whether there is an afterlife. It would serve no purpose to challenge him.

We were already within a day of death, and he was firm. Half-heartedly I had rehearsed every one of the arguments that had won our skirmishes over the previous eight years. They were our old friends now, and we spoke of them gently, without recrimination. Larry knew I was speaking for my own conscience, and he listened politely. He even smiled at the idea of dying in the electric chair.

'It's got no fear for me now, Clive,' he said. 'You think about dying on the Cross. Days of suffering, dying from thirst. At least it'll be over in a few minutes. I can deal with it.'

I almost believed him.

I had written up voluminous pleadings that we could file if only he would authorise it. But we all knew now that, even with his consent, the odds were long. At the last hearing, Judge Camp had made sure that Larry waived every possible right.

I had to be at the prison by six for Larry's sake. He had asked me to witness his execution. His sister, Chris, asked me to go too. She was afraid of the stories she had read. They could do anything to you in those last few moments. There had to be someone there on Larry's side to intervene. Many months back I had let Larry down when I could not summon up the courage to be there. Now, my emotional reserves were back up.

My wife Emily and I pulled into the truck stop on the way to the prison as I did not have a mobile then. The phones were ranked next to the toilets, with Larry's stereotypical tobacco-chewing Southerners, all truckers, passing by me as I called the office in Atlanta. Larry was on the line. He wanted to talk to me, and they patched us in on three-way.

'How're you doing, Larry?' I asked, the banal American greeting.

'You can file that thing, Clive,' he said in a calm voice. I was silent on the other end of the line. What was Larry saying? 'Why don't you just go ahead and file that thing you've been working on, Clive?' he repeated. 'You got my permission.'

Larry had changed his mind again. I was elated to be back fighting, however long the odds. I thanked him – what other word could I use? – and passed the phone to Emily to carry on talking. I immediately called Mary Beth Westmoreland, and then Judge Camp. Soon we were having an argument by conference call, and I was struggling for Larry's life from a dimly lit bank of telephones in a filling station, lowering my voice as the truckers in their overalls passed by towards the men's room.

When we left to go on to the prison, Emily recited her conversation with Larry.

'What'd Clive look like when I told him he could do it?' had been Larry's first question. Emily had cautiously explained how happy I had been to lower my lance to tilt at the windmill once more.

'Good. That's good.' She could imagine his smile at the other end of the telephone. 'I planned it this way. I wanted to let him try once more. I know it's too late now, but it's kinda like saying thank you, I guess.'

And it was too late. I still had the law on Larry's side, and got the better of the final argument to Judge Camp, but we all knew that Larry had vacillated once too often. The Eleventh Circuit and the Supreme Court were each prepared for a final flurry of appeals, and did not pause in denying them.

I reached the prison in time to have a final conversation with Larry on the telephone from the visitors' area.

'You don't have to be there, if you can't do it,' Larry said. I had confessed how I just could not do it the last time.

'No, Larry, don't you worry about me,' I said, with more confidence than I could have mustered up the year before. 'I wouldn't let you be alone, without a friend. Not now.'

'Well, Clive, you have been a friend,' Larry said, his voice flat but almost ethereally calm. I could feel him choosing his words, a final speech he wanted to make. 'You know, you stuck by me. And I'm real grateful for it. I couldn't have dealt with this last year, the year before. I can now. Back then, I was afraid. I'm not afraid now. Not at all. I'm ready for it. And that's thanks to you. Even before I learned I was worth something, even before I learned that from Jesus, you let me know you thought so. Maybe it's been frustrating for you, but you helped me till I was ready. I want you there tonight, if you can. 'Cause you've been my friend.'

He was through. I felt as though I was being strangled. I stared at the yellow prison wall in front of me. I looked up at the ceiling, the white tiles. I wanted to deny it. I had put him through years of suffering. But I could never deny that I had been his friend. I had always meant to be his friend.

'I'll be there for you, Larry. I wouldn't be anywhere else.'

That was all I could manage.

'See ya then,' said Larry. 'Bye for now.'

His voice never wavered through our last conversation as the hour approached. And he never wavered in the chamber.

Larry had given me his lotto numbers. He still thought there was a chance he might be able to manipulate them. It was, in a way, the ultimate honour – he wanted my charity to benefit from the tens of millions he might win.

I put a bet on. Not even one number out of seven came up. Maybe the preachers are right, and God really does disapprove of gambling.

After the prison killed Larry, they wanted to get rid of his personal effects. I took the pitiful bag of papers that made up his entire bequest. In it was a copy of a letter to Wanda, the daughter of Margaret Sweat, whose death had been recorded on the telephone:

I hope this letter finds you and your daughter well!

I received your letter. I was planning on writing you before I died. I had already had a friend get your address for me. I'm enclosing it (typed address) to prove what I just stated. Also, you left off your house number on your envelope (see enclosed).

The reason why I didn't want to tell you before now what your mother's last words were was because I knew it would just cause more pain to you, another reminder of your mother's death. But I realise now her last thoughts and words would also bring some comfort to you as they showed how much she loved you.

Wanda, even though your mother knew she was going to die, she was more concerned about you than herself. She begged me not to kill her because she had a daughter. Her exact words: 'Larry, please don't kill me. I have a daughter.'

I'm crying now, after writing the preceding paragraph.

I can't put into words how sorry I am for killing your mother and the Smiths. I ask you to forgive me, not for my sake but for your sake, because if you are a real Christian you have to. Please read: Matthew 6:14–15; Mark 11: 25–26; and Luke 6:37.

In closing, I can't reiterate enough on how sorry I am that I took your mother from you and the grandmother from your daughter.

You are in my prayers!

Love,

Larry

PS 'Life can't be lived with bitterness. That feeling defeats the human spirit. Life should be lived in the shining, healing light of hope and forgiveness.' – Nelson Mandela.

How Larry! I thought. Tidying up loose ends in the kindest way he could imagine, both for her peace of mind and to protect his family.

31

The Death of Dad

Does the road wind up-hill all the way?
Yes, to the very end.

Christina Rossetti, 'Up-hill'

It was shortly before Christmas 2006. Dad was in Addenbrooke's Hospital after a heart attack. Mary flew in from Australia at once. There was a sense that this could be the end. I was back living in the UK, partly to be close to my ageing parents, so I had come up to Cambridge.

The NHS doctors and nurses were providing Dad with an incredible service. He was in a little private room. His back was giving him pain, and the encroaching dementia was more obvious than ever. I spent a couple of hours a day sitting by his bed – it took my first visit to work out how to handle it. He was not up to any kind of coherent conversation, but then I printed off a number of his favourite poems. I would give him the first line, and he would quote them. As I listened and prompted, I pondered how each spoke to him and of him. Dad loved the natural beauty of the world around us, and would stop to take in a 'view' whenever we were driving somewhere in my youth – that was Wordsworth's 'I wandered lonely as a cloud'. Rossetti's 'Up-hill' – 'Of labour you shall find the sum' – was his obligation to leave his mark on the world.

Shelley's 'Ozymandias' was the paradox. Many poems battle for primacy in my own life, but perhaps 'Ozymandias' wins out, solely because it is my most direct link to Dad. He used to recite it, with just the right emphasis on each grandiose syllable:

that 'shattered visage . . . whose frown / And wrinkled lip, and *sneer* of cold command / Tell that its sculptor well those passions read / Which yet survive . . .' When I later analysed it, I wondered whether Dad read this as the working-class pretender to the world class of Cambridge. Yet to me it was Dad's voice. It was his love of the words rolling off the tongue. Shirley Bassey aside, Dad never really listened to music; yet the music of language stirred his unconquerable soul, as Henley put it in 'Invictus'.

By now, he had an automatic response to anything, from someone coming into the room or pulling out sheets of poetry: 'Thank you very much.' His autopilot was, in the end, one of gentle good manners. I would stroke his forehead. My mother used to do it to me when I was unwell, and it is the most calming experience in my world. I hoped it had the same effect for Dad. 'Thank you very much,' he said.

A patient in the next room was being told how to use a walker. 'Thank you very much,' Dad said.

Ultimately, though, I wanted to sense how Dad felt towards what seemed inevitable, since I knew we were close to having to make a decision with or for him. I read to him a stanza by Thomas Hood, from one of his favourite poems.

I remember, I remember,
The house where I was born,
The little window where the sun
Came peeping in at morn;
He never came a wink too soon,
Nor brought too long a day,
But now I often wish the night
Had borne my breath away!

I did not ask him directly, but I wanted to know how he was feeling towards 'the undiscovered country from whose bourn no traveller returns' – whether he was OK with it. Whether he still felt that he was a traveller who would return. The best I could do was ask him how far we should be asking the doctors to take his treatment.

He looked at me, directly in the eye, and for the first time in days I felt he was truly speaking to me. 'I'd like to stay with you,' he said. It was clear to me that Dad wanted to hang on for as long as he could. He was not, it seemed, ready to find out the answers.

When Mary arrived, we alternated beside his bed, as it was a personal time. Mary and I did have one very incoherent conversation with him together, when he would speak long sentences about the car being in the right place. Mary brought up the stud, thinking he would respond better to the distant past. He reacted to the names of stallions including Psidium and Hook Money, but when she asked him to describe his most precious animal, Forlorn River, he seemed stumped.

25 November 2006 was a Saturday. Dad had a catastrophic heart attack. His heart stopped, tired out from working at full speed for eighty-one years. Somehow they got it going again. Those doctors were astounding.

Mary and I were riven. We had not set a DNR (do not resuscitate). It was the mirror image of Larry – he had wanted to die, and I had stopped him. Now Dad had told me he wanted to hang on, but he was in terrible pain. I was keeping something of a diary at the time. Wednesday 29 November: 'After meeting with the doctors, I wrote up the letter that is essentially Dad's death warrant. It was not difficult to find the right words – I am a lawyer, after all, and it was just an exercise in ensuring that I wrote what we really meant, while leaving room for their medical judgement. But after I had finished writing, the true impact of what we were doing struck me and Mary, as we talked about it.'

We had just overridden Dad's express wishes. However certain the conclusion seemed, it was very hard. He was in pain all the time. The best the brilliant medical staff could do was to neutralise it, in which case he was essentially comatose. Dad had always been about the quality of his life, and he had virtually none. Yet I had been having the closest relationship of my life with him. The assumption that we had the right to choose for him was enormous.

Mary and I delivered the letter to the young doctor. When we next visited Dad in the hospital, we noticed that there were now no monitors for his vital signs. We realised that this was something we had brought about. Matt, the Australian doctor, told us that there would be a new elderly care team who would be coming to assess him and take him on. At first, I was confused, as another doctor had said, just two days before, that they would be the point of contact for Dad for the foreseeable future. Matt seemed embarrassed and did not try to explain; Mary probably understood at once, but it took me ten minutes to figure out that there was now no reason for the cardiac care unit to remain on his case.

Dad was a little brighter that morning, which made me feel particularly guilty. He was feeling nauseous and needed a bowl. 'Thank you for being so good to me,' he said. I read him various poems, and he perked up for 'Up-hill', where he got a couple of the lines right, including the last line, 'Yea, beds for all who come.' He responded particularly to 'She Walks in Beauty' by Byron. He seemed to appreciate having his head stroked.

A few days later I had to give the annual Longford Lecture, on prison reform. I tied it into Dad's situation, and that made me break down. It was a little like giving a closing argument at the penalty phase, but this time angling for death.

Three days before Christmas was Mum's eightieth birthday. It was overshadowed by Dad being in hospital, which seemed unfair – she had done so much more for us, when all was said and done. Dad was just hanging on. Mary had to get back to Australia and her family.

On 15 January 2007, the doctors decided Dad was stable

enough to move to a palliative nursing home, rather than continuing to take up a hospital bed. It would need to be one with end-of-life care, so he could not go back to the warm and friendly place in Ely, where his room had already gone to another person. He was moved into a new nursing home on the outskirts of Cambridge. The next day, a Tuesday, Mum and I went to visit. We could see the place from the bypass. When we took the next exit, it was more difficult to locate than it had seemed. After one wrong turn we made it to a parking area to the side of a front entrance that resembled a cheap American motel. As we went in, the atmosphere was immediately oppressive. We never got as far as seeing Dad's room as they brought him in his wheelchair to the front hallway, rather like the prison visits I had at the Georgia State Prison in Reidsville all those years ago. The staff bore an air of heavy harassment. Dad looked up, shrunken, from his chair, marginally with us. Further down the hallway, one of the other residents was letting out an animal howling.

I vowed to get Dad somewhere else when I got back from my trip.

I was in Nouakchott. A few weeks back, I had never heard of the place; I certainly could not have spelled it. Not so long before that it had been a small village, chosen to become capital to the newly independent Mauritania, a country twice the size of Britain. Nouakchott had swollen to nearly a million. I was representing Ahmed Abdel Aziz, one of three of their citizens in Guantánamo; his family was well connected.

I received the news of Dad's death as I got back from a trip out towards the vast expanse of the Sahara. I spent half an hour looking out of the window of my hotel at the black sky. Air France were surprisingly unhelpful. In the end, I could change my flight only because Ahmed's brother-in-law was a minister and came to the airport with me. Then the stewardess spilled red wine all over my one suit and, when I asked what we could do about it, she brusquely told me to go wipe it off in the toilet. All in all, it was a slightly disastrous trip home.

By the time I got back, Mary was already making arrangements to come over again. With typical efficiency, she was planning a slide show of pictures of Dad's life for the memorial service.

On Wednesday 31 January, Mary and I went to the funeral home to see Dad one last time before the cremation. It was near the bottom of Duchess Drive, the steep mile of towering beech trees from the main gate of Cheveley Park Stud. How many times had we passed by, every day to Fairstead House Primary School?

I don't understand the world of the British undertaker. In New Orleans, the Second Line funeral is a singing and dancing celebration of the life of the person going to the grave. In England, the experience is a dirge, with grey people whispering. Mary and I went past the faux decor to the back, where we each took our turn with the open casket. Dad was pallid, with just a hint of the stubble that roughed my cheek as a small child. He was waxen, though he looked more at peace than he had for much of his life.

'Dad,' I whispered, 'you should know that you have made a wonderful life possible for me, for which I will be forever grateful.' I am not sure I had ever cried over Dad before. 'I am so sorry that I failed when it came to you. But I love you, Dad. For whatever that is worth now. Goodbye, Dad.'

My mother drafted a brief obituary for the *Newmarket Journal*:

Richard Stafford Smith, born in Newmarket on 30 August 1925, died after a brief illness on 22 January 2007. Richard was the son of Albert and Trix Smith, and brother of Jean Malins. He attended the Perse School in Cambridge. He was still underage, at only sixteen, when he volunteered to serve in the RAF Pathfinders during the

Second World War, being promoted to the rank of flight lieutenant. After the war, he took a degree at Corpus Christi, Cambridge, in Estate Management. Richard married the former Jean Thomas, of Fordham, on 9 July 1955. They had three children, Mark, Mary and Clive. After a spell employed by the university, he took over the running of Cheveley Park Stud upon the death of his father in 1958, continuing until 1972. His second marriage was to Dawn Snelling on 2 November 1979 (later divorced), with whom he had a daughter, Kate (now Bedford). For many years he lived in Spain, returning to live in Cambridge and then Ely, where he later enjoyed help from the exceptional staff at Vera James House. Richard was cremated after a memorial service at the West Suffolk Crematorium, organised by Southgates of Newmarket. Parallel memorials were held by family members in Canberra (Mark and family) and Townsville (Mary's family), in Australia. The service was taken by Rev. Tony Winter, an old friend from All Saints Church, Newmarket, who gave an address entitled 'Faith, Fun & Fellowship'.

There was a smiling picture of Dad on the front of the order of service, the way I would want to remember him. There was nothing about 'Dick' – it was all either 'Dad' or 'Richard'. He told nobody until he was eighty, in Vera James House, that he had always hated being called Dick. The poems ('I Wandered Lonely as a Cloud' and 'Up-hill') were the obvious ones – we left 'Ozymandias' for another day.

The service ended with the Beatitudes from the Sermon on the Mount.

Blessed are the poor in spirit, for theirs is the kingdom of heaven.

Blessed are they who mourn, for they shall be comforted.

Blessed are the meek, for they shall inherit the earth.

Blessed are they who hunger and thirst for righteousness, for they shall be satisfied.

Blessed are the merciful, for they shall obtain mercy.

Blessed are the pure of heart, for they shall see God.

Blessed are the peacemakers, for they shall be called the children of God.

Blessed are they who are persecuted for the sake of righteousness, for theirs is the kingdom of heaven.

32

An Epitaph

I regard the brain as a computer which will stop working when its components fail. There is no heaven or afterlife for broken-down computers; that is a fairy story for people afraid of the dark.

Stephen Hawking

KRYTEN: It's the electronic afterlife. It's the gathering place for the souls of all electronic equipment. Robots, toasters, calculators. It's our final resting place.
LISTER: I don't mean to say anything out of place here, Kryten, but that is completely Whacko Jacko. There is no such thing as 'Silicon Heaven'.

Red Dwarf, 'The Last Day'

Of Dad's bequests, the one I value most is an unwillingness to view accepted dogma as the objective truth delivered by a god on tablets from Mount Sinai. One term I don't like is 'mental illness', let alone the way we apply it as a society. I would like to see us do away with the whole concept.

I do not pretend this is my original idea. The 1978 Basaglia Law initiated the closure of all Italian psychiatric hospitals. Named after Franco Basaglia – the leading Italian psychiatrist of his time – there were multiple motives behind the law. There was the perception, which surely my great-grandmother Frances Canham understood, that such asylums were designed effectively to ostracise the 'mentally ill' from society, as our forefathers did lepers.

And there were the notorious cases: psychiatrist Giorgio Coda, while never imprisoned, was prosecuted for torturing people. Coda believed that negative conditioning would cure 'defects', and he used electric shocks (which he dubbed 'electro-massage') to 'cure' alcoholics, drug addicts, masturbators and homosexuals, though sometimes they died in the course of it. He assumed this would stop their conduct, as Pavlov conditioned his dog. (To be sure, the torture of my Guantánamo Bay clients can stop them from telling the truth.) Most people would agree that Coda was an extreme example, and yet we still use electroshock treatment without really understanding how it works – or even what we are curing.

Meanwhile, the way the term 'mental illness' is thrown around is emotional torture for many, including my father.

One of the ameliorative goals of the Basaglia Law was to cut inpatient figures, thereby integrating people into the local community where possible, and taking regular hospital admissions only upon necessity. Over ten years, from 1978 to 1988, the rate of inpatient care fell by almost two-thirds.

Parallel experiments were also taking place in other countries – with mixed results. The United States might seem like a success story: the number of people institutionalised has dropped by 90 per cent since the 1950s, down by over half a million. This masks an ongoing catastrophe. There was a recognition that those deemed 'mentally ill' should be treated rather than merely warehoused, but another stated objective was simply cost-cutting. Efforts to limit institutionalisation resulted in many erstwhile patients being rendered homeless. Harsh laws, including the criminalisation of homelessness itself, have created a sad reality today: there are more than three times as many people classified as 'mentally ill' in US prisons than in psychiatric hospitals.

Globally, another development that has helped patients get out of asylums is the increased use of psychiatric medicine. Who, one might well ask, could be opposed to using medicine as an alternative to a psychiatric hospital? Who could be opposed to alleviating suffering with a simple pill? I once suffered an anxiety attack, and was immensely glad that I was able to knock my pointless, swirling thoughts firmly on the head with lorazepam.

While all of this is true, psychiatric medication is often used without understanding what we are medicating, or without grasping the underlying causes of what we have deemed the 'illness'. This is well illustrated by the haphazard way we started using haloperidol to treat schizophrenia – as experienced by my fifteen-year-old death row client Troy Dugar. The same can be said of the lithium used to treat bipolar disorder.

Meanwhile, despite the good intentions, Italian practice stalled. It seems to me – from a lifetime observing my father, my clients and myself – that there are some irrational orthodoxies (beliefs?) which might be hampering our understanding. If we reconsider them, perhaps it will let us focus our efforts towards Dr Basaglia's original goals.

While I have used the term 'mental illness' with inverted commas in this book, I would rather telegraph my distaste for the phrase: first, we overuse the word 'illness'; and second, it manufactures a distinction between 'mental' and 'physical' illness.

When addressing a physical illness or disability, our approach is by and large reasonable: we treat what needs treating, and push society to accommodate differences. We would not dream of criticising you if your mother took thalidomide during pregnancy. We would not blame any disabled person for their misfortune, even if a horse rider was paralysed when unwisely taking a dangerous jump. We generally show sympathy. We build ramps for wheelchairs (the Americans do it better than the British), and we hold alternative Olympics that do not require someone with one leg to compete against someone with two.

There are, of course, limits to our good sense with physical issues, as there were when we blamed lepers for their illness and put them in colonies. Regardless, we lag far behind in our approach to 'illness' or 'disability' that we deem psychological. If your mother drank too much alcohol when she was pregnant with you, you may be hyperactive, have a bad memory and show lack of attention in school. As a result, you are likely to be classed as a bad student, or just plain lazy. We label this foetal alcohol syndrome (FAS), but we still approach it very differently from the 'thalidomide child'. FAS is not currently 'curable', so it makes little sense to call it an illness – it is a condition. We should make accommodations for those with the condition, but we should not expect them to show more than an incremental change in behaviour – any more than the 'thalidomide child' can grow another limb (though we hope one day we will make that possible).

Equally, the *DSM* differentiates personality disorders from other diagnoses in a way that is distinct from our approach to physical issues. Dad's supposed narcissistic personality disorder was deemed to be distinct from his bipolar disorder. Yet the very idea of a personality disorder strikes me as simultaneously too narrow and too broad. The definition of antisocial personality disorder is so broad, for example, that while prosecutors use it to send many of my clients to death row, it is equally applicable to many lawyers, hedge-fund managers and members of the British cabinet: they are self-centred people focused on personal gain. Ultimately, we must ask why we chastise people for their 'personality disorder' when it is just the way their temperament has been shaped.

At the same time, the categories of 'personality disorder' are also too narrow: why do we not include a simple diagnosis of 'lazy' in the manual? I am a self-confessed workaholic. I never sat down and decided to have that personality, any more than a kid has a seminal moment in his childhood when he decides to lounge around and watch television all day.

We might look at all such 'personality disorders' slightly differently, and see most of the 'traits' or 'temperaments' as no more, or less, than a part of each person's humanity. Each individual is built up in a complex way. We can elect positively to encourage one behaviour over another – altruism over self-aggrandisement, for example – but when best-laid plans fail, we should not start disparaging people as 'skivers' rather than 'strivers'. Rather, we should look to maximise each individual's happiness by both understanding them and helping to channel them so that they maximise their contribution to society.

Looking at my father, he had a very particular personality. For the most part, it does not make sense to label him 'ill', though he needed help on the occasions when he was depressed. In retrospect, at least, we can see that he could have been channelled much more effectively than he was – by the mad careers advisers who thought he would fulfil his life as a factory inspector. He had brilliant and original ideas, but there were two primary flaws in his interaction with society. One, he had been brought up to think he was going to be judged primarily on how much money he made, and yet he was ill-adapted to such a task – and hence he always saw himself as a failure, which would edge him towards the depressive end of his nature. Two, he was hopeless at implementing his ideas because, due to his 'mania' (for want of a better word), he was always running after the next shiny object. His life worked moderately well so long as my mother was there for him to lean on for help. After her, he never had another partner who could fulfil this role.

I recognise all this in myself. I am fortunate that I have never encountered his black dog, but I am still my father's son. I avoid the accumulation of money as a goal in life, because I witnessed what it did to Dad. Tilting at the windmills of government injustice is a much better psychological fit, as there are plenty of ways to bat away my own self-criticism. It is true that Edward Johnson would likely be alive today if I had known in 1987 what I know now, and in that sense there is no escaping my feelings of guilt. However, I am under no illusion that he would be alive today had I opted simply not to take his case: the deplorable state of the legal system meant that he had no better option.

Had Dad been steered to this kind of career, he would have had a good chance of happiness. He would have loved the endless arguments, and he would have excelled in them. He would have taken joy in what seems a pure moral stance. He could have worked all day and most of the night, without harm to anyone. If he had a novel legal argument, the worst that could have happened was for the courts to reject it.

Given his character, he would still have needed help with 'facilitation'. Sometimes people tell me they sift through the concepts I have – some they think are good and some are not. With notable exceptions, I disagree with this. I believe (perhaps arrogantly) that most of the ideas could benefit our clients. However, I accept that I am sometimes unrealistic about what can be achieved with limited resources. Understandably, there is not a cadre of people out there whose temperaments are suited solely to helping to turn my dreams into reality. Thus, even as I write this book, I am failing to do justice to a number of projects, and thereby letting down some victims of human rights abuses. So I muddle along – in my case, imperfectly but nevertheless with great job satisfaction. Dad could have done the same, but he would have needed to be recognised for who he was, and to see it himself, and to have someone to help him move his ideas onwards.

Even after the bankruptcy of the stud, Dad's happiness could still have been salvaged in part had I helped to set him on a path towards his other passion – poetry. This could do little harm and give him much satisfaction. Had he wanted to be a poet all his life, society would have had to provide a welfare system of sorts (just as it would if I wanted only to write books that did not sell in sufficient numbers to earn a living). Perhaps it will be a while before we recognise the need for a guaranteed minimum standard of living, but we will get there one day. That, and permission to write poems, would have maximised the chance that Dad would have been happy.

The world was not created to satisfy Richard Stafford Smith & Son, however, and I use the two of us only as examples. The same rules apply to everyone else. Ultimately, instead of insulting each other, we should celebrate our differences. Indeed, we might take Alain de Botton's advice to discuss openly how each of us is 'mad'. (The word is, of course, pejorative and I am sure he would agree to substitute a gentler term – perhaps we could discuss our 'idiosyncratic tendencies'. The essence is that we need to encourage insight into what they are.) We should spend our energies trying to understand people (and ourselves), to work out how best to mesh temperament, strengths and passions with the world.

When we dream, some accuse us of airy-fairy idealism. Let us not be insulted by that. If we do not have a faraway goal, we will not know which way to travel. (It makes little sense, to give just one example, to expect to get closer to the utopian ideal, shared by many, of a world without prisons, by incarcerating more people.)

However, there is a very real world out there, with which we must deal every day. Larry Lonchar had a 'temperament' that was, in many ways, like Dad's. He lived in a very ugly world. Those who like to despise others will tell us that he was a murderer, the lowest of the low. I knew him for many years and beg to differ. Regardless, there was nothing I could ultimately do to prevent his execution, when faced with the combined forces of a hateful world and Larry (who hated himself). I did not have the power to create a life for him that was even moderately acceptable. Under these circumstances, sometimes a 'solution' that seems unpalatable is the only one, as Larry taught me in a very stark way.

I have known children who have loved their terminally ill

parents and yet have helped them to die – my sister and I did that for our own father, even making the decision for him. I have known parents who have loved their tortured and depressed children so much that they have gone along with their deaths as well. If we are not clever enough to cure cancer or to overcome depression, then for now in rare instances that may be the only realistic avenue open to us. Nothing can be harder, but I have only respect for those whose love extends to taking some of the pain onto themselves.

Larry's grotesque death was in some ways comparable. It was a very human moment. Just as many people may have no compunction helping a terminally ill person take her own life with opiates if she wants it, so Larry's conversion to a sincere Christianity was a wonderful gift to him that I accidentally facilitated. We can be disgusted at the society that would treat Larry in that way, but in the spectrum of options that were available to us, the dignity of his death was perhaps the best we could hope for.

Larry was certainly grateful, and that is what matters most.

What is it that compels us to differentiate between 'mental' and physical illness? We once thought that physical illness was linked to the 'humours' of the body, and this led us to all kinds of unhelpful 'cures', like bloodletting. Today, we continue to come up with odd distinctions between the mind and the body.

Dad was obsessed with religion, reincarnation, the 'soul' and 'free will'. But we don't need a delusion that there is a unique human 'soul' to inspire us to find our existence extraordinary – any more than I need the implausible promise that I will one day play cricket for England to allow me to enjoy a match with the Mapperton Marauders. It should not diminish our sense of marvel at highly complicated creatures evolved through millions of years. As mentioned earlier in the book, one of my colleagues jokes that I am half-robot, half-machine. I am fine with that, but humans (and other animals) are of such fascinating physical and emotional complexity that I, for one, would have to live through many of Dad's reincarnations before I would begin fully to understand my 'robotic' self, let alone anyone else.

While we recognise that our mental well-being is linked to our physical health, and vice versa, we often still think of them separately. Would it not be more sensible to accept that our 'mental' health is just a part of our physical health? Would this not help the way we approach seeking remedies? Some things often do not need a cure; with others, any cure is currently beyond our ken; but in either case, we would not blame the patient.

If the distinction between mental and physical seems an irrational one, it also has many dangerous consequences. Inevitably, the logic of all this turns us to the very issue of responsibility and punishment. Suffice it to say here that while we move rather rapidly towards a gentler educational approach for our children, we insist on punitive measures for strangers. I do not plan to embark on an exegesis here on the folly of prison, yet surely we can agree that we should treat the children of others as we treat our own – and not merely until an arbitrary time when they attain eighteen years of age. It is not such a radical notion: religious traditions have implored us to 'love thy neighbour as thyself' for at least 2,000 years.

In law school, my professors indulged in lengthy debates on the foundations of our right to punish people. Is it deterrence? Is it the individual's revenge? Is it society's retribution? Is it incapacitation? Is it 'rehabilitation'? For the most part, I found these discussions academic and pointless since surely our goal should be to treat others how we would like our loved ones to be treated. Most of us would like our children to be educated and socialised; we do not wish to see them executed, whipped or incarcerated.

The dogma that insists on responsibility and punishment

carries with it many unhelpful consequences, including the adversarial process that condemned Larry Lonchar. Doctors were paid large sums to quibble over whether his suicide by electric chair was 'rational' when surely the lowest threshold of civilisation would have insisted that we turn to the Samaritans to get him help. Some countries are taking tentative steps towards 'restorative justice' which focuses on understanding on both sides. That must surely make sense.

In this regard, we cannot expect to achieve nirvana any time soon, but it seems fairly obvious which direction we should take. We should aim to be kind, both in our actions and in our interpretation of others. It is not always easy, but the alternative is much harder on us, and on those around us.

Dad often preached Thomas Paine:

These are the times that try our souls. The summer soldier and the sunshine patriot will, in crisis, shrink from service; but one who stands up deserves the love and thanks of all. Tyranny, like hell, is not easily conquered; yet we have this consolation with us, that the harder the conflict, the more glorious the triumph. What we obtain too cheap, we esteem too lightly. Heaven knows how to put a proper price upon its goods.

ACKNOWLEDGEMENTS

I want to emphasise that this is my version of history, not that of my siblings (Mark, Mary and Kate) and I appreciate their forbearance in letting it be so. I wish I could thank Larry Lonchar, and his family; that he could think to be generous to me just before Georgia killed him in the Electric Chair helped to turn a nightmare into a moment of humanity.

I never give enough credit to my brilliant agent Patrick Walsh, who labours along with John Ash and Emily Hayward-Whitlock, treating me like a real writer as opposed to the amateur that I indubitably remain. (Patrick actually read the first draft, which was a War-&-Peace 250,000 words; both publisher and reader owe him a debt for encouraging the removal of about 60%.) Quite why Kate Harvey and her assembly at Harvill Secker continue to be so positive about my ruminations I have no idea, but I should thank at least Mikaela Pedlow, Tom Atkins, David Milner, Kate MacDonald, John Garrett and Oliver Grant.

I cannot omit my 95-year-old mother Jean for all she has done, including her unwavering support for my father even after she had the good sense to divorce him, and for saving all the memories upon which I could draw. Also my wife Emily and son Wilf for putting up with me as I worked through both the book and the concomitant therapy. As ever there are many people to thank, and I hate the inevitability of forgetting people. I will conclude by acknowledging the readers, and I welcome a discourse on the important issues that I have tried to cover in this book.

CLIVE STAFFORD SMITH is a lawyer specialising in defending those accused of the most serious crimes, and is founder and director of the UK non-profit 3DCentre, as he was previously with legal charity Reprieve. Based in the US for twenty-six years, he now works from the UK where he continues to defend prisoners on Death Row, and challenges the continued incarceration of those held in secret prisons around the world. He has secured the release of 81 prisoners from Guantánamo Bay and still acts for six more. His book *Bad Men* (shortlisted for the 2008 Orwell Prize) described this campaign. His second book *Injustice* was shortlisted for the 2013 Orwell Prize and the CWA Non-Fiction Dagger. Alongside many other awards, in 2000 he received an OBE for humanitarian services.